────GINS

How ginseng has been used as a panacea for thousands of years in the East; its natural habitat, and cultivation of the root throughout the world; some scientific evidence of its properties; its effect on the ageing process; the different forms available, and dosage; its future in the field of medicine.

About the Author

Stephen Fulder is a biochemist and experienced medical research scientist with specialist knowledge in the field of complementary medicine and in particular in Chinese herbal medicine. He is a distinguished expert on ginseng and has written and lectured widely on the subject.

GINSENG
The Magical Herb of the East

STEPHEN FULDER, MA, Ph.D

THORSONS PUBLISHING GROUP ·

First published as *About Ginseng* in 1976
This completely revised and
expanded edition published 1988

Ginseng root used on the front cover supplied by The Korean
Ginseng Centre, 108-110 Charing Cross Road, London, WC2.

British Library Cataloguing in Publication Data

Fulder, Stephen
Ginseng. — Rev. and expanded ed.
1. Medicine. Herbal remedies: Ginseng
I. Title   II. Fulder, Stephen. About
ginseng
615'.32368 7

ISBN 0-7225-1619-3

Published by Thorsons Publishers Limited,
Wellingborough, Northamptonshire, NN8 2RQ, England

Printed in Great Britain by
Richard Clay Limited, Bungay, Suffolk

3 5 7 9 10 8 6 4 2

Contents

—Acknowledgements—

I would like to acknowledge Joseph Needham for the use of his library, and Helen Varley and Arthur Rashap for comments on the manuscript. Of course I would also like to acknowledge the help of ginseng, without which this book would have taken much longer.

CHAPTER 1

Brother of Soma

Of all the multitude of plant medicines known, ginseng may claim to be one of the most interesting. It is a plant which, for thousands of years, has been uniquely regarded as a panacea — a universal remedy. Its full name, *Panax ginseng,* illustrates this, for Panax, like panacea, comes from the Greek word for 'all-healing'. No other plant is used so widely in the Orient for so many diseases and ailments. The Chinese, whose traditional medicine is without doubt one of the most sophisticated medical systems known to man, rely heavily on ginseng both as an essential tonic and restorative and as a regular part of the complex battery of plants compounded for the treatment of serious diseases.

Ginseng is unique because it is the plant used most widely in combating some of the degenerative conditions and loss of vitality that accompanies ageing, and, not surprisingly, a special reverence for it has developed over the ages. It is embodied in many stories and legends; in fact, it could be said that no other plant has such an extensive mythology.

There are other unique features of ginseng which are important for our point of view: It seems to be a plant which is very typical of traditional oriental medicine. If we can unravel some of its subtleties it will tell us about the medical system which gave it birth. Certainly no other has been the subject of such extensive scientific research yielding such paradoxical conclusions. Finally, it is strikingly obvious that there is no other medicinal plant which is so widely respected in one half of the world, and so misunderstood, and even scorned, in the other half.

The Ginseng Plant

Panax ginseng is the botanical name of the Asian ginseng plant, given to it by the botanist and explorer Carl Anton Meyer. It belongs to the small family called the _Araliaceae_ which it shares with, among others, the spikenard and the ivy. For such a famous plant it has remarkably humble herbiage. It has arrays of five serrated leaves atop a long, straight stalk which may be 20-80 cm tall, depending on age. The older plants may have two or more of these stalks. There are pale green flowers which only begin to appear when the plant is two or three years old. These produce bright red berries which are well-liked by birds, as by humans. The birds spread the seeds, which are the size of a small lentil.

The medicinal part of ginseng is under the ground. It is the root, which is fleshy and thick somewhat like a yellow carrot, although it has many tendrils and rootlets and may sometimes be branched, curled or bent. At the top of the root is a crinkled 'neck', which is, in fact, a short underground stem which bears the buds for each season's growth. The fresh root tastes somewhat bitter, with a hint of an aromatic sweetness.

Ginseng is a deciduous perennial. That is, the above-ground foliage dies off every autumn and the root lies dormant, sleeping under the cold winter ground, often thick with snow, until the dormancy is broken in the spring. One or more buds on the neck sprout new stems which emerge in April or May. The flowers spread in June, the seeds ripen in August, and the foliage yellows and dies by October, leaving the root ready for another winter dormancy. Each annual cycle leaves its mark — a wrinkle on the neck above the root. The age of the plant is thus easily counted by the number of its wrinkles.

The home of the Asian ginseng is the high temperate forests of China, Korea and the Eastern USSR. However it is now virtually extinct in its wild state. At the same time cultivation has now spread the 'domesticated' ginseng to many other areas in Eastern Asia.

Ginseng Relatives

The closest cousin to the Asian ginseng is the native species of North America, described botanically as _Panax quinquefolium_. It looks very similar to the Asian ginseng, though a little more compact, and it is also famous as a medicine with the North American Indians. The resemblance between the two species is expected. Chinese flora and fauna, including the medicinal plants, are closely matched on the other side of the Pacific. *Panax quinquefolium* is cultivated in China anyway, and it grows in the Himalayas.

There are other Panax species, all of which are used in traditional medicine, though none with the same reputation. *Panax pseudoginseng* has a short fat root and seven leaves, more narrow than those of ginseng, leading to its Chinese name 'jen-seng San-ch'i' (Three Seven Ginseng). It grows in China, especially in Yunnan. There is a Japanese variety of this species. Then there are a small group of Himalayan relatives scattered throughout the forests of Nepal, Sikkim, Bhutan, Tibet and Assam. There is one plant, however, which is not related to ginseng though some have mistakenly claimed it to be. That is the mandrake. It may have a man-shaped root like ginseng, but botanically it is not even a distant relative, and medicinally it will knock you down not pick you up.

Ginseng as Legend

A medicinal plant as important as ginseng may be more than just a medicine to the people who use it. It is sometimes seen as a veritable gift from the benign divine powers. Extensive ritual can surround the gathering, planting, storing, preparing and consuming of the root. The many legends have given rise to many names. One story describes how the village Shantan, in Shensi province, was troubled for many nights by a groaning and wailing somewhere behind the village. Although much afraid of this strange occurrence, the villagers organized an expedition one night to discover the source of the unearthly cries. They took torches and staves and eventually localized the sound to a large bush about a mile away. They dug up the bush and found underneath a huge root, of the shape and size of a man. The crying stopped. From this the root became known as 'spirit of the earth' (*ti ching*).

Ginseng is derived from the words *jen shen,* which means a crystallization of the essence of the earth (*shen*) in the form of a man (*jen*) or more simply, 'man-root'. The same word also means 'like-the-constellation-of-Orion'. Orion is traditionally shaped like ·

a man, and is also the constellation which has astrological influence over ginseng. Other names of ginseng are: blood-like (*hsueh shen*), human bridle (*jen hsien*), devil cover (*kuei kai*), magical herb (*shen tshao*), and the more down-to-earth name, the-regenerating-elixir-that-banishes-wrinkles-from-the-face (*tson mien huntan*). The Koreans call the herb Korean phoenix (*Poughwang*). The Japanese are more prosaic with their word: 'Korean carrot'.

The Man-like Root

The Chinese undoubtedly revere the wild ginseng, now unfortunately almost extinct, above any other plant. They also regard ginseng, even if cultivated, as probably their most important medicine. This respect is reflected in the fabulous prices that were paid for the wild root during imperial times. An old wild root, cured properly and of the best quality, would fetch much more than its weight in gold, giving rise to the sarcastic epithet in Manchuria: 'Eat ginseng and ruin yourself'. It was believed that the power of a plant to cure a certain part of the body was reflected in some ways in its form. Thus a ginseng root that was shaped like a man was believed to have greater curative powers for the whole body, and particularly for the restoration of male potency. Even today such a wild root will fetch thousands of dollars among the Chinese communities overseas. This is also the cost of a treatment with wild ginseng in Korea today, for those lucky enough to find a traditional practitioner who possesses such a rarity.

Manchuria is the traditional home of the most famous wild ginseng. The Manchurians boast that 'the weeds of their country are the choice drugs of the Chinese'. It is often mentioned that one Chinese Emperor set out to war in order to capture ginseng-growing land, and it is certainly true that in 1709 the Emperor sent 10,000 Tartars to search for ginseng, ordering that each soldier should give him two catties of the best and sell the rest for its weight in silver. The Chinese sometimes used to keep the ginseng in lead-lined boxes, carefully wrapped in silk and tissue paper, for they believed that it had certain 'life-giving radiations' which might be lost in an ordinary container. Such radiations are in fact unlikely, but it illustrates the reverential and almost sacramental treatment given to the herb.

In China the general opinion was that ginseng was the prince of plants. The most famous Chinese herbalist, and one of the founders of Chinese traditional medicine, the Emperor Shen Nung, put forward a classification of herbs which is recorded in the Shen Nung Pen Tshao Ching, the *Pharmacopoeia of the Heavenly Husbandman,* printed in the second century BC. Several hundred herbs were listed. Ginseng is at the top of the list of those agents which are beneficial, yet harmless.

Ginseng in India and Korea

China is not the only place where ginseng has been used since ancient times. The Vedas are ancient Indian scriptures which reflect an oral teaching which may be 5000 years old. The Atherva Veda has many hymns describing ways to attain health and fulfilment. One hymn describes ginseng as 'the root which is dug from the earth and which strengthens the nerves'. It continues: 'the strength of the horse, the mule, the goat, the ram, moreover the strength of the bull it bestows on him. This herb will make thee so full of lusty strength that thou shalt, when excited, exhale heat as a thing on fire.'

The hymn then describes the herb as 'brother of Soma'. Soma is the legendary life-giving plant of India, an elixir which was worshipped and offered in sacrifices. If ginseng is the brother of Soma, it must also have appeared to have unearthly power. On the other hand, ginseng is not a feature of the Ayurvedic medical system which developed out of the Vedas. This may be because the plant later became unavailable in India.

Wherever it grows, ginseng has given rise to its own myths. In Korea, it is related how a son and grandson, both very poor, were devotedly looking after an ailing grandfather. One night the grandson couldn't sleep. The candle kept on blowing out. He was suddenly aware that there was no wind to blow out the candle and that there must be a spirit presence in the room. The boy took a needle and thread, and the next time he felt the presence of the spirit he plunged the needle in that direction. The needle disappeared and the boy followed it by means of the unravelling thread. Eventually he found the needle. It was stuck in the ground at the base of a wild ginseng plant. The boy took the plant and brewed a decoction for his grandfather, who recovered. Thus the spirit of the ginseng plant had rewarded the boy for his selfless devotion.

There are many more myths and rituals, some of which will be related when discussing the way ginseng is collected and cultivated, cured and consumed. The essence of the legends is that ginseng has an almost supernatural power for the good of man. We can understand this a little better if we consider the Chinese philosophy of the Tao. The Tao literally means 'the way'. It is the incomprehensible flow of energy of the cosmos which finds its temporary expression in the materials of nature. Man is also made of these materials, and he will be healthy if he achieves harmony with the Tao, the essence of the world. Ginseng was imagined to contain all the elements necessary to adjust the body of man in tune with nature. If man were in greater alignment with nature he would have more of its strength and energy, therefore it could have a profound effect on health if used wisely. Ginseng represents a beneficial aspect of nature and this is why it is treated as such a great gift.

CHAPTER 2

Ginseng and Herbal Medicine in China

You exist on plants. Virtually all the food that you eat is either from the plant kingdom, or from animals who eat from the plant kingdom. The number of different types of plants in use as medicines is certainly greater than all the plants in use for any other purpose. The Indian system of traditional medicine, the Ayurvedic system, said to date from 3000 BC, holds that not a single plant in the plant kingdom is useless. Plants are blessed for the help they give. As it says in the Vedas:

> All the many herbs in which the human physicians
>   find a remedy,
> Like mothers assembled let them yield milk
> Unto man, for freedom from harm.

Many plants, such as digitalis, raowolfia, datura and ephedra, are used exclusively for medicines; others — for example, those commonly known as garlic, mint, coffee, banana, caraway and liquorice — are both food and medicine. In Chinese, as in western natural medicine, there is anyway little difference between a food and a medicine. The path to health involves all the substances consumed by and connected to the human organism.

Compare this with the naïve view of herbal remedies held by most conventional doctors. Dr Williams, working in China at the turn of the century, writes cynically about Chinese traditional medicine: 'Anything indeed that is thoroughly disgusting in the three kingdoms of Nature is considered good enough for medicinal use.' Dr Williams also appears to have come to the conclusion that almost every plant is useful in medicine, although he refuses to see it as a blessing.

Conventional medicine has rid itself of the traditional plant remedies during the early part of this century, describing them as unproven and uncertain concoctions fit, perhaps, for grandmothers to dispense but not doctors. None are now left in the official western pharmacopoieae, or lists of acceptable drugs. They were discarded without ever being tested to see whether in fact they could achieve the results that traditional practitioners, and patients, claimed for them; it was the fashion for chemicals, the emerging pharmaceutical industry, and the creed of scientific medicine that banished the plants, rather than the evidence of their ineffectiveness. Modern medicine thereby reduced its options to stronger chemical drugs. Only now, after many years of concern and alarm at the pervasive side-effects of such drugs, is there a renewed interest in those mild plant remedies and medicinal foods that were left by the wayside. Plants such as aloes, comfrey, garlic, feverfew, chamomile or liquorice are slowly beginning to be reinvestigated.

The medicinal resources in the plant world are enormous, most of them completely unknown to science. It is reliably estimated that science has investigated less than one per cent of the plant species for medicinal activity. Traditional medicine has, in contrast, developed through thousands of years of experience, of observation and experiment. It knows which plants to use, for what purposes, how and when to use them, in what combinations, and for which types of person.

A Kingly Herb

Chinese traditional medicine is probably the most complicated and esoteric medical system known, and little of it is properly understood in the West. We can return to the *Pharmacopoeia of the Heavenly Husbandman* to find an interesting clue to the way herbs were used in China. Those which are mild in effect and not harmful, even in large doses, are the 'kingly' herbs, for example, ginseng, liquorice and jujube (Chinese dates). The second group, more powerful herbs which are rather more toxic, are called 'ministerial'. The lowest group, called merely 'adjutant', are the highly powerful herbs which are at the same time dangerous. These include aconite and hellebore.

The essential point is that the mildest herbs are the most

important and of the first rank, while the really powerful herbs are the last-resort drugs to be used only when the others fail. This is of course the opposite position to that of western (allopathic) medicine, which regards the powerful drugs as the mainstay of medicine, and the mild drugs as accessories of little significance.

The basic principle of Chinese traditional medicine is to attempt to maintain the body in peak health. If the body is healthy it will automatically be more resistant to disease, just as a car which is tuned and serviced will be much less likely to undergo a serious breakdown. Therefore the primary task of the traditional practitioners is to ensure the continuing health of the people they look after, and secondarily to treat diseases. A Chinese doctor used to be paid by his patients only when they were in good health. When they became ill the doctor was not paid, because he had failed to keep his patient healthy. It is fair to say that while the focus of traditional medicine is on health, the focus of allopathic medicine is on sickness. We can now see why the mild herbs are the most important, the 'kingly' ones. They are the first and primary weapon of the practitioners in health maintenance, and ginseng is among the leaders of the kingly herbs.

Superimposed on this fundamental concept are complex instructions which relate different herbs to different kinds of disturbances within the body functions. For example, the body, as all nature, consists of active, male, expanding, burning or 'yang' qualities and passive, female, contracting, conserving 'yin' qualities. These qualities must be in equilibrium for health, an equilibrium which takes into account the kind of constitution that a person has, and the yin and yang forces in the foods, the weather and the general environment. Ginseng is extremely yang. It is taken in Chinese medicine when organ systems are too yin and sluggish. The effect is to burn up wastes and increase the flow of energy in an organ system.

The yang, energizing nature of ginseng is well understood by oriental practitioners, and used as a guide to when and how to take ginseng. Thus it is most useful in states of health where energy is depleted and the body has slowed down. This indicates its special virtue in cases of tiredness, exhaustion, convalescence and advanced age. It is, by the same token, not effective where someone is vital, young, energetic and awake.

Another key principle of Chinese medicine is called the five elements. These are descriptions of the texture and constitution of natural processes, similar to the early Greek elements of earth, air, fire and water. The Chinese elements are described as wood, fire, earth, metal and water. These are poetic metaphors which refer to forces or processes in nature. Earth for example, implies solidity, and fire, activity. Health requires a proper relationship between the elements in the body and those in the external world. If the body is too 'watery' it is susceptible to cold and damp diseases such as those of the joints. Ginseng, as a root of man, is described as benefiting and harmonizing all the elements. However the Asian ginseng is regarded as predominantly a heating remedy and therefore beneficial in conditions where the body is cold or watery. For this reason it is understood that:

1. Ginseng is best used to increase health and prevent disease in the autumn and the winter, and not the summer.
2. It is helpful to prevent and treat 'cold' diseases, including those of poor or inadequate circulation, elimination or digestion, weakness, metabolism and sexual activity.
3. It is better used in colder climates.
4. It will be arousing, stimulating or 'heating' to the brain.

American ginseng, though similar in many respects, is not heating. Therefore the Chinese say that it can be taken in the summer and is preferable in hot climates. It is also not so arousing or stimulating. Indeed people do find it to be, if anything, slightly sedative.

Traditionally, an oriental remedy is rarely used alone. The Chinese have developed a wonderfully sophisticated method of building combinations of plants which help each other. If a stronger remedy, such as *Rehmannia glutinosa,* is used to stimulate an organ, in this case the kidney, it is combined with others such as *Alisma plantago* to quench or disperse the heat created by the former medicine's action; in other words to remove waste and protect the organ while treating it. If *Ephedra* is given to promote sweating and clear out a cough and cold, cinammon may be added to help the circulation, and apricot seed to promote the coughing up of phlegm, which *Ephedra* would otherwise prevent. Liquorice would be added to combine all the ingredients, to remove poisons and protect the stomach. Three quarters of all Chinese medicines contain more than four ingredients.

Ginseng is one of the most frequently used of all oriental remedies. It is present in more than a quarter of all the classical prescriptions. However if we divide oriental remedies into those that are adjustive, preventive and restorative, or 'kingly', and those that are more directly curative, we will find ginseng in the majority of the tonic remedies. It is also a component of quite a few mixtures for more serious diseases, such as of the circulation or nervous system. In these cases ginseng is not usually the curative backbone of the recipe. It is more likely to be there to support the energy and vitality of the patient while the other plants help against the disorder.

There are so many formulae in use containing ginseng that a classical authority, Chieh-pin Chang, published a book in AD 960 listing more than 500 formulae containing ginseng. They covered nearly every type of disease, with few exceptions.

A common general tonic, for example, is made up as:

Ginseng extract	2 parts
Root of *Atractylis lancea*	2 parts
'Fou ling' (*Pachyma cocos*)	2 parts
Liquorice (*Glycyrrhiza uralensis*)	1 part
Ginger	1 part
Red Jujube dates (*Zizyphus jujube*)	1 part

It is a tonic mixture developed by Li Shih Chen, China's most famous herbalist of the seventeenth century.

The 'Vital Essence' formula is:

Lycium fruits (*Lycium chinensis*)	2 parts
Schizandra chinensis	2 parts
Ginseng	1 part
Deer Antler	1 part

This is said to build the male hormones and increase virility and energy. A typical recovery tonic, used to return to health quickly after a disease, increases energy, gets rid of poisons and improves the metabolism:

Ginseng	3 parts
Wild Asparagus root (*Asparagus lucidus*)	5 parts
Schizandra chinensis berries	5 parts
Rehmannia glutinosa	2 parts
Ligusticum lucidum	2 parts
Tree Peony	2 parts
Bitter Orange Peel (*citrus aurantium*)	1 part
Liquorice (*Glycyrrhiza uralensis*)	1 part

Other components of mixtures can augment the effect of ginseng in subtle and quite remarkable ways. For example liquorice will direct the action of ginseng to the metabolism, and strengthen the immunity, *Cimifuga heracleifolia* will focus it on the lungs, and *Poria cocos* directs ginseng to the kidneys. Ginger is described as a servant that helps ginseng warm and strengthen the body, and orange peel spreads its effects evenly throughout the body.

───────────Chinese Medicine Today───────────

Traditional medicine in China is not an archaic code of instructions present only in old books. It is a living system which is used today in combination with allopathic medicine in a unique synthesis. For example, in the teaching hospitals of Peking, surgery will be carried out in the western manner with highly advanced equipment, but the anaesthetist may use acupuncture instead of pentothal, and herbal preparations will be used for pre- and post-operative treatment. Ginseng is often present in these preparations to increase the resistance of the patient, protect his system against shock during the operation, and increase his vitality during the post-operative recovery.

Western medicine came to China during the last century. Hospitals and clinics were built and traditional medicine suppressed. However, during the revolutionary wars, traditional medicine proved invaluable and was reinstated alongside western medicine after the revolution. Rural health workers, the famous 'barefoot doctors', taught sanitation, and gave vaccinations in the villages, while the traditional practitioners gave acupuncture treatment, herbs and massage.

Traditional medicine then spread to the cities, where it is now studied at research institutes. In this way the Chinese hope to extract the best from 4000 years' worth of experience in herbal medicine and acupuncture. The Chinese have not succeeded in understanding ancient principles in scientific terms. However, they have proved that traditional medicine works, whether or not it conforms to the current scientific theories. If Chinese herbal medicine is judged with a 'proof of the pudding' attitude, one cannot fail to be impressed. As an eminent pharmacologist, Dr Lewis Lasagna, remarked on a visit to China: 'We may look forward to a whole range of new drugs of enormous potential for medicine in general.' Ginseng is the first of these.

The Uses of Ginseng

The *Pharmacopoeia of the Heavenly Husbandman* states that ginseng is a 'tonic to the five viscera, quieting the animal spirits, strengthening the soul, allaying fear, expelling evil effluvia, brightening the eyes, opening the heart, benefiting the understanding, and if taken for some time, it will invigorate the body and prolong life'.

More modern pharmacopoeias (manuals of medicines) echo this earliest record. They state that ginseng alleviates tiredness, headaches, exhaustion, amnesia, and the debilitating effects of old age, and confirm that it is a useful adjunct in the treatment of tuberculosis, diabetes, diseases of the heart, kidneys, nervous and circulatory systems. It is said to prevent declining potency in older men. A more modern Chinese text, for example, states that it is used for anyone with general weakness, including 'those with signs of anaemia, lack of appetite, shortness of breath accompanied by perspiration, nervousness, forgetfulness, thirst, lack of strength and lack of sexual desire.' In other words, though it is not a cure for specific diseases, it is regarded as a powerful restorative agent, which has effects that are not limited to any organ or tissue, but are spread throughout the body.

Its ability to increase general vitality is what makes it so precious in the eyes of the Chinese, for they regard vitality as the essence of health. This is why it is one of the most important Chinese medicines. At the same time, the breadth of the oriental claims made for ginseng has confused westerners. The oriental herbalists saw that ginseng increased vitality and heat, making available an added source of energy to diverse organs, and therefore helping in a large variety of health problems. Westerners wrongly assumed that one remedy that assisted in so many conditions must be a panacea, and gave it its name, *Panax*. Since a panacea is an ultimate consumer product, advertisers took up the message and touted it as a cure for every disease you could think of. Ginseng, an essential tool for maintaining and improving health to orientals, became to westerners a cure-all and therefore a joke. Indeed oriental medicine does not even have the concept of a 'cure-all', it is more concerned with 'all-health'. Even the Greeks, who originated the word Panacea, were thinking of health, not healing, since the word is the name of the goddess Panacea, known as the goddess of complete health rather than complete cure.

A Stimulant

It is traditionally held in all the countries which use ginseng that it is a stimulant and can increase the resistance of the body. The sick take it to restore strength. Chinese soldiers carry it on to the battlefield to prevent the effects of stress and shock if they are wounded and to sustain them until they can be brought to the field hospital. Soldiers also use it as a stimulant for sentry duty, and it is recorded that the North Vietnamese used it extensively in the recent war.

After a series of experiments at the Soviet cosmodrome, Soviet experts in space medicine concluded that ginseng was a better stimulant or tonic for their cosmonauts than amphetamine drugs such as dexedrin, used by the U.S. astronauts. It increased their alertness and performance more successfully than the amphetamines, without a consequent hangover, and it didn't prevent proper sleep and rest. Cosmonauts took ginseng and related plants with them on space missions in the 1970s.

A similar situation pertained with Soviet sportsmen. After a long series of trials, particularly at the Lesgraft Institute of Physical Culture and Sports, the director, Professor Korobøv, concluded that the action of ginseng-like plants should be 'aimed at accelerating the restorative processes after intensive activity, and at increasing the body's resistance to unfavourable external influence.' The result was that Soviet sportsmen were instructed to take ginseng, or a Soviet relative *Eleutherococcus*, to help overcome exhaustion and stress during training. They also use them in sports events, including the Olympics, to gain access to the last ounce of energy.

The stimulant action of ginseng is graphically described by Father Jartoux, the French priest who brought it to the notice of the Royal Society of London, by means of a letter published in 1714. Whilst surveying the area of the Chinese border with Korea, a local Mandarin gave him some ginseng which he took. 'In an Hour after I found my Pulse much fuller and quicker, I had an Appetite, and found myself much more vigorous and could bear Labour much better and easier than before.' Later, he was riding with the Chinese emperor until he was so exhausted that he could hardly keep himself from falling off his horse. The Emperor gave him half a root of ginseng. He chewed it, whereupon he forgot all about his tiredness and carried on full of energy.

The plant can save the lives of seriously ill patients by giving them the energy, vitality and stamina to fight the disease. The Chinese have described many cases in which the sick have been practically *in articulo mortis* when, upon administration of good quality ginseng root, they have been sufficiently revived to carry on items of business. It is a common practice in China to give ginseng to someone on his deathbed in order to give him the power to receive his family and arrange his affairs before departing this world. As Dr Porter Smith noticed: 'Several cases in which life would seem to have been at least prolonged by taking doses of the drug so as to allow intelligent disposal of property, indicate that some positive efficacy of a sustaining character does really exist in this species.'

Such comments are not limited to Orientals. For example, Dr Whittie, a Fellow of the Royal College of Physicians, in the seventeenth century, was given some ginseng while at Hull, in England, and used it on a patient who was

'much emaciated, and reduced into a perfect Skeleton, a meer Bag of Bones, by a long Hectick Feaver, joyned with an Ulcer of the Lungs; being despaired of by all Friends, I was resolved to try what the Tincture of This Root could doe, which I gave every morning in Red Cows Milk, warm from her Duggs. And I found his Flesh to come again like that of a Child, and his lost Appetite restored, and his natural Ruddy Complexion revived in his Cheeks

to the Amazement of his desponding Relations, that he
was called 'Lazarus the Second'.

Ginseng has also earned itself a reputation as an aphrodisiac
(a drug which stimulates sexual desire). In fact, *Encyclopaedia
Britannica* uses ginseng as an example of a 'genuine' aphrodisiac.
There are many records of its use by Chinese Emperors and
their court in order to maintain the required Imperial virility, a
symbol of the health of the Empire. Many of the oriental tonic
remedies are concerned with the maintenance of sexual energy,
partly because in oriental culture this is seen as a crucial sign
of overall good health. Ginseng is often combined with other herbs
and exotic materials such as sea horses, deer horn, and various
animal organ extracts, for this purpose. This has, not unexpectedly,
caught the imagination in the West. Ginseng will certainly be
found in sex shops and it occasionally turns up in the media, as
the subject of waggish comment. Indeed this has led most of the
public to view ginseng as 'some kind of aphrodisiac'. In actual
fact it is not an aphrodisiac, that is a specific sexual stimulant,
and the Chinese do not claim this for it. Indeed even the extent
of its oriental use for this purpose is uncertain. While the Emperors
are known to have consumed much ginseng at court, they
probably took it as a general tonic to improve their overall vitality
and vigour rather than as an aphrodisiac per se. It may be that
its reputation as an aphrodisiac owes much to the fancy of
European observers at the Imperial court rather than to fact.

A somewhat similar mistake may have been made in describing
it as an aphrodisiac as in describing it as a panacea. The quite
remarkable property of ginseng is to increase deep vitality and
energy. One of the results of improving the access to this energy
may well be increased sexual virility. But another result will often
be increased memory and mental function. And just as you cannot
describe it as a cure-all because of its positive effects on overall
health, you cannot properly call it a memory-drug nor an
aphrodisiac because of its positive effects on overall human
performance.

On the other hand, ginseng is used very widely to combat
impotence, especially the decline in virility which occurs with
age. So much so, that Dr Jeffries, in his *Diseases of China,* observes
that ginseng is used 'chiefly in cases of matrimonial unpro-

ductivity'. He seems to have been struck by the popular use of ginseng for that purpose, rather than by any of its other multitudinous uses. Travellers in China, from Marco Polo onwards, have also been impressed by the virility of the Chinese people of advanced years, and the Chinese themselves readily admit that it is partly the use of ginseng which is responsible.

Long-term Benefits

The herbal tradition of ginseng states explicitly that the more ginseng is taken, the more long-term benefits can be obtained from it. It is recommended that everyone who can afford it should take a course of ginseng every year. The effect is cumulative. The regular use of ginseng, it is stated, will not only increase health and vitality but will also prolong life. Old people are advised to take some every single day to extend their lifespan and to encourage protection from the diseases of old age. If it can be authenticated that it is really a 'regenerative elixir that banishes wrinkles from the face', it will be the first known medicine or drug which would be specifically useful for the aged. We devote a subsequent chapter to this intriguing possibility.

Other oriental countries which use ginseng as part of their traditional medical system ascribe properties to it which are almost identical. The *Materia Indica* of 1826, for example, states that ginseng 'nourishes and strengthens the body, stops vomiting, clears the judgement, removes hypochondrias and all nervous affectations, and in a word, gives vigorous tone to the body even in old age.'

When ginseng was first brought to Europe its special ability to improve vigour in the aged, and therefore perhaps to increase lifespan, was particularly noted. As one seventeenth-century English doctor writes: 'Public Fame saith, that the Popes of Rome, who are chosen to that Office when they are very Old, doe make great use of this Root, to preserve their Radical Moysture and natural Heat, that so they may the longer enjoy their Comfortable Preferments.' While William Byrd, a Fellow of the Royal Society and author, noted that though it did not appear to be useful in 'Feats of Love', it gives 'uncommon Warmth and Vigor to the Blood and frisks the Spirit, beyond any other Cordial . . . it will make a Man live a great while, and very well while he does live. And what is more, it will even make Old Age amicable, by rendering it lively, chearful and good-humour'd . . .'

The Uses of American Ginseng and Other Ginseng Relatives

American ginseng, *Panax quinquefolium,* is very close to Asian ginseng botanically, it is exported in large quantities from America to Asia, and it is often regarded as equivalent to Asian ginseng so that the word ginseng covers both without differentiation. This confusion of species has damaged ginseng's reputation, for the august Smithsonian Institute tested the American ginseng and finding it ineffective as a stimulant, declared that all ginseng is worthless. But are they equivalent? Are the traditional claims made for it the same as those for Asian ginseng?

Panax quinquefolium is regarded by the indigenous peoples of North America, who discovered its use there, in a manner similar to the Orientals and their ginseng, but with less hyperbole and veneration. They do not regard it as the chief of their medicines. They describe it as an aid to digestion and appetite, and a help against cramps and menstrual problems. The Creeks for example, would drink an infusion of the root for exhaustion, breathlessness and croup. Other tribes describe it as a supportive aid for the wounded. The Cherokees, in a similar vein to the Orientals, describe their ginseng as 'the little man' and acknowledge it as a tonic. Clearly the Indians understand its support for the energy and metabolism, but they do not use it as a stimulant or rejuvenating plant.

In China, where both roots are available, the traditional view is that American ginseng is *yin* while Asian ginseng is *yang.* It does improve the function of the organs, by balancing the flow of their metabolism rather than speeding it up. It is therefore taken to improve health, energy and resistance. Interestingly, its predominantly yin 'female' quality makes it more suitable for women to take whereas Asian ginseng is more suitable for men. For a similar reason it is used in preference to Asian ginseng in hot climates or during the summer months. As it is a sedative rather than stimulating tonic it is used by people who need vitality but are already constitutionally yang, that is active, agitated, nervous or hot. For such people the Asian root might create excessive stimulation and the American root can help build their strength and allow proper rest. In general, however, good quality Asian ginseng, if available, is usually preferred to the American species.

Of the other ginseng species only *san-ch'i* ginseng, *Panax pseudoginseng var. notoginseng,* is a mainline traditional medicine. It is a weak tonic and its main use is to disperse unwanted blood in the body, for example in bruises, swellings, internal bleeding and irregular menstruation. The Himalayan tribes and Indian doctors use the Himalayan relatives of ginseng as minor medicines in cases of poor appetite and weak digestion.

CHAPTER 3

The Root that Hides from Man

Yet another of the names given to ginseng is 'The Root that Hides from Man'. This is meant literally, for the root prefers a habitat deep within thick forest, in moist, rich and undisturbed soil. It sometimes favours specific trees as neighbours, as this Korean song shows:

> The branches which grow from my stalks are three in
>   number, and the leaves are five by five,
> The back part of the leaves is turned to the sky, and
>   the upper side downwards,
> Whoever would find me must look for the Kia tree.

Finding wild ginseng was so difficult that searchers could do little else but pray to the spirits which guard it to favour their quest. In Korea, wild ginseng gatherers would keep chaste and pure for a week before the expedition, praying continuously to their guardian deity. The team was always a group of ten senior villagers led by 'The Man'. They used a secret sign language during their quest, and would refrain from talking, for they were fearful of incurring the displeasure of the Nature spirits guarding ginseng.

In China it is related that searchers were assisted because the leaves of the ginseng plant would sometimes glow at night. The glow would go out if anyone approached, so the searcher would shoot an arrow at it and come back in daylight to look for the arrow and pull the plant. The glow has led to some extravagant theories concerning supposed radiations from ginseng. However, it is more likely to be glow-worms or moonlight reflected from the leaves.

Most of the gathering of wild ginseng in Manchuria used to

be done on behalf of the Emperor. The common people had to try poaching, or make do with inferior cultivated or imported roots. A few plants still grow wild in Manchuria, the Ussuri region of the USSR and in Korea, but extensive picking and the felling of forests have more or less dried up the supplies of the wild root in the East. No more than a kilo or two of genuine wild roots are dug every year in the whole of Asia, and these roots are likely to fetch thousands of dollars each when they find their way to the market. There are still sufficient stocks of wild American ginseng, *Panax quinquefolium,* to yield about 100,000 lbs a year. However, it has now been declared an endangered species and its export is regulated by the US Government.

Ginseng Cultivation

The earliest plantations of ginseng were in south-east Manchuria, and in North Korea, and cultivation is still carried out in those places, though the product is entirely for home consumption. Major cultivation areas have developed in China, South Korea, Japan and the USSR. There are United States consular reports which describe how the Russians started their ginseng plantations in South Siberia with young plants worth 120 million dollars which were taken home from North Korea in the aftermath of the war. The USSR has wound down ginseng cultivation in the last 25 years in favour of other Araliaceous plants.

Cultivation in Asia is big business. For example it earns South Korea about a hundred million dollars annually. Yet it is still carried out with ceremony and elaborate preparation. Prayers are said before sowing. The seeds are sown into specially prepared germination beds in the autumn, one year after they are collected. They need the intermediate year, or more precisely, the cold of an intermediate winter, to get ready for germination, and they need the second winter to complete their dormancy time. They germinate in the spring and grow one year in their seed beds. After the first year of growth they are normally transplanted to new beds with appropriate spacing. In Asia they may be transplanted at least once more before harvest. Harvest will be at the fourth, fifth or sixth year, in the autumn, when the above-ground parts are yellow and dying off, and the root has collected the most nutrient.

Cultivation of ginseng requires very well drained, clay-based, loamy soil containing organic matter, such as leaf mould. The field should preferably face north and slope gently. The plant does not need a great deal of fertilization or manuring as it is slow-growing, but the earth should be slightly acid (pH 5.5). Shading is required, to mimic the natural deep-forest growing conditions. Korean research has shown that the plant grows best with shade that only lets 20 per cent of the light through. In Asia the shading is provided by rolls of straw matting that is spread on frames over the bed. The beds should also be heavily mulched with leaf litter or other materials such as straw.

Ginseng is difficult to grow because of all the pests and diseases, especially fungi, which affect it in the close confines of intensive cultivation. Traditional methods, developed over 400 years in Asia, protect the plant by frequent transplanting to fresh beds, and by never using beds for growing ginseng that have had ginseng on them within the 12 previous years. However this has not proved practical today when there are considerable pressures to grow ginseng in ever-greater quantities on an ever-diminishing supply of suitable land. The last few years have seen up to a third of the Asian ginseng crop affected by disease.

Against this background, there is the US cultivation of American ginseng. 800,000 lb. wt. of ginseng (*Panax quinquefolium*) is now grown in North America, about the same as the Japanese ginseng production. This compares to three million pounds weight in South Korea and two-and-a-half million in China. American ginseng is today grown with a high level of agrotechnical expertise despite the fact that most ginseng is grown by family farmers who have switched from milk or potato production. Plastic shade net is used, and in contrast to Asia, the farms are mechanized. The roots are not transplanted during growth although they may be thinned, and disease is dealt with by extensive spraying with agrochemicals. Asian countries are under pressure to compete and are phasing out their traditional organic methods in favour of modern agricultural methods including sprays against disease.

Ginseng in America

The American *Panax quinquefolium*, though not trumpeted as a panacea or elixir of life, was still a most useful folk remedy. The

Shamanistic Indian tribes in the mountains of mid-America used it with more ritual, sorcery and spirit guidance than the scientifically minded Chinese taoist herbalists of the time. Naturally in the colonial period, ginseng was wildly advertised by the notorious quack doctors of the early white settlers in America, but so was everything else. The official United States Pharmacopoeia during the last century did list ginseng as a stomachic and stimulant.

The ginseng grown in America provides an extraordinary story from an economic and social point of view. It is not commonly known that ginseng digging provided the main source of support for some of the early settlers in America. The enterprise began in Canada where a Jesuit missionary, Father Lafiteau, discovered in 1716 a plant similar to the one described by Father Jartoux in China. Avid collection soon began for despatch to China, which was an unlimited market for ginseng, and boatloads were exported to Canton at a profit so huge that ginseng became second only to the fur trade in profitability.

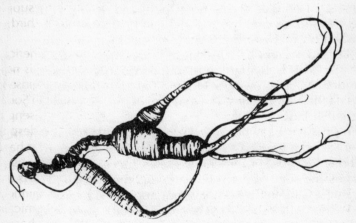

A 41-year-old wild American ginseng root.

────────End of the Canadian Trade────────

Indiscriminate picking and inadequate preparation of the roots dried up the Canadian trade by 1760. The United States took over, and trade expanded. In 1862, a good year for the trade, 622,761 pounds of dried roots were shipped to Canton and Hong Kong. Fur trappers used to return from the mountains with fur and ginseng, and in fact ginseng trade in America today is still carried out by the fur companies. Entire villages in Kentucky and Wisconsin used to go out into the forest and, with 'mattock and sack', dig for 'seng', as it was known. They sometimes managed to collect bushels of roots in a day. The price rose and rose. It is recorded in a book on Daniel Boone that he personally collected large amounts of ginseng and purchased more from the white settlers. In the winter of 1787-8 he started up the Ohio in a boat containing nearly *fifteen tons* of ginseng. The boat overturned and he lost it all. Undismayed, he had collected fifteen 'caggs' again by the following autumn.

When wild ginseng became scarce at the end of the nineteenth century, some enterprising farmers attempted cultivation, and a few made a great success of it. However, as we have seen, ginseng is liked by other species besides humans and glow-worms — namely, all kinds of insects, fungi, pests and worms. Virtually the entire American crop was wiped out in 1910, and the Depression finished off many farms. Despite this, cultivation continued in the US and it is now a flourishing industry worth some $50 million per year. This is centred on Marathon County, Wisconsin, with additional crops growing in Ontario, Canada and throughout the Appalachian Mountains. The majority of this ginseng is exported to the Far East.

Has ginseng been grown in Europe? Father Lafiteau sent fresh samples from Canada to France, where they were transplanted without success. Yet ginseng is grown successfully in research centres and state farms in Bulgaria and the Ukraine. The Royal Botanical Gardens in Kew have not attempted to grow it. There is no reason why it should not be grown in Europe and other places, yet there is no report of anyone having done so. Here is a golden opportunity for someone with green fingers!

Ginseng in the Market

The root which is available in shops is never fresh. It has undergone an elaborate process of curing and drying which preserves the essential medicinal components and allows the root to be kept for years without decay or decline in potency. The dried root is hard and has a strong aromatic bitter-sweet taste.

After carefully digging the root from the earth, the fine outer tendrils are removed and it is washed. Some of the roots are steam cured by a secret process which turns them a deep red colour and gives them a remarkable translucent appearance. Others which are not steamed are yellow and opaque. Slow drying in a sequence of warm rooms at different temperatures for a period of months finally preserves and hardens the root and it is ready for consumption.

The steaming process is intended to preserve the root more effectively, and proof of this exists in a red root placed in the Royal Storehouse of Shosin in Nara, Japan, by the Buddhist priest Kan-Jin in AD 756. It is in good condition and laboratory analysis has demonstrated that it contains all the chemical constituents expected of it. Only the best quality roots, grown in certain areas, are steamed in this way. Poorer quality roots tend to develop soft centres if they are steamed. For these reasons the treated red roots ('red ginseng') are held to be of better quality than yellow roots ('white ginseng').

The quality of the Asiatic root varies considerably. This is to some extent reflected in the price, which is also set by world demand. First quality is the wild Asian ginseng which is hugely expensive and never seen outside the Orient. There is some old cultivated Asiatic ginseng, such as Chinese 'tassel' ginseng, which is next in price. Then comes the majority of cultivated roots, and their price and quality vary with age. Asian red ginseng is usually of higher quality than white because only the older and better roots are selected for the special processing. Japanese red or white ginseng is generally regarded as inferior to Chinese or Korean. It is not possible to compare American and Asian ginseng as to quality because their medicinal properties differ, the Asian being more arousing and heating (yang) than the American, which is more relaxing (yin) in its tonic action. Wild American ginseng is much more expensive than any of the cultivated roots, in both East and West. Care should be taken when purchasing ginseng to ascertain its origin.

Ginseng is now a major world crop, valued by the International Trade Centre of the United Nations at over $200 million at

wholesale prices. This would put it at around one billion US dollars
at shop prices, after it has been made into products. '. . . ginseng
currently represents one of the largest currency earners among
medicinal plants', comments the International Trade Centre. In
the Far East and among oriental communities in the West, ginseng
roots are sold as they are, singly or in boxes of 600 gm. The price
paid is dependent on quality, size, age, region of growing and even
shape, the more man-like the root the better. However ginseng
is processed into tablets, capsules, instant teas, and other products
for western, and increasingly also young Asian consumers. By the
time the ginseng is on sale in the shop in, say, capsules, its price
may be five to ten times that of the original dried roots.

The commercial potential of ginseng is also changing official
attitudes to it. Fifteen years ago westerners were completely
dismissive of a medicine that all Orientals regarded as their most
potent. Indeed this strange fact aroused my curiosity, and in 1971,
first tempted me to start research on ginseng. Today the puzzle
has been partly resolved, for the public are not so ignorant of
ginseng, and experts are prepared to at least tolerate it, though
few understand it. It is now in the Soviet, Japanese and Asian
pharmacopoieas, the official lists of drugs, and it is one of the
few plants left there. More than that, it has just entered the Swiss
pharmacopoiea, the only new plant to do so for many years.
Entries in the pharmacopoieas of other western countries will
probably occur in the end. This is mostly because ginseng has
been so visible in pharmacies for so many years that the authorities
cannot help putting it in the official drug lists, if only so as to
help pharmacists distinguish the real thing from its substitutes.
Once this has happened, it would be correct to state that ginseng
is here to stay.

The high cost has always encouraged fraudulent substitutions
of other roots for ginseng: for example, *Campanunoea pilosule,*
also called 'Bastard Ginseng' (*tang shen*) in China, and *Adenophora
verticillata (shashen)* both resemble it. In America red dock root
has sometimes been sold as red ginseng. The Chinese relate a
traditional method of telling the real from the fake. Two people
are chosen and made to walk four Li (a Li is the Chinese mile).
One has a piece of the supposed ginseng in his mouth. If at the
end of the walk the person without the root is somewhat out of

breath, while the man with the root does not feel in the least bit tired, then the drug is true.

There is another plant which has come into the limelight indirectly as a result of ginseng. The Institute of Biologically Active Substances in Vladivostok, USSR, attempted to find substitutes for ginseng because of its rarity and its reluctance to take to cultivation, searched through the *Araliaceae* family and discovered a range of stimulatory and adjustive remedies. The most effective and safest was a common thorny shrub called *Eleutherococcus senticosus,* which grows in Siberia, China and Korea, and had similar medicinal properties to those of ginseng. Tests showed that the roots and leaves possessed wide-ranging tonic effects, and *Eleutherococcus* has become widely used in the USSR and officially recognized by the health ministry as a restorative. It is given to athletes, cosmonauts, factory workers and those who are highly stressed, convalescent or debilitated. However, little knowledge exists of *Eleutherococcus* outside the USSR. In Chinese medicine it is called *ciwuja* and used somewhat like ginseng, though it is not so strong. The continued interest in *Eleutherococcus* stems from its wide availability in the wild. Factories in the Far Eastern provinces of the USSR now extract *Eleutherococcus* on a large scale and distribute millions of doses every month. It has become known as Siberian ginseng, or *Eleuthero*, although in fact it is far from ginseng botanically. Nevertheless it carries some of the kudos of the true ginseng and at a quarter of the price, *Eleutherococcus* is a popular second string.

CHAPTER 4

Some Scientific Evidence

The Chinese herbals and the Chinese medical tradition give only a brief mention to the fact that ginseng is a stimulant and will overcome exhaustion. They concentrate rather on the long-term usage in the restoration of health and vitality. Subtle long-term effects on health are difficult to measure with the techniques of modern science, so that research has concentrated more on detecting short-term actions. This has emphasized the stimulant effect of ginseng in the eyes of westerners, but it must be remembered that the emphasis in traditional and herbal medicine is just the reverse.

Yet scientific research has shown ginseng to be an effective short-term stimulant, and this is of great potential interest to westerners, who are badly in need of a stimulant which does no harm. Ginseng, on the contrary, may be a stimulant which actually is good for you, depending on your state of health and functioning.

Some of the earliest experiments on this stimulant action were carried out on mice by Professor Brekhman, head of the Institute of Biologically Active Substances in Vladivostok. He devised a swimming test to see if ginseng could increase stamina. Mice are put in water, where they swim until they are exhausted. They are allowed to rest, and then made to swim a second time. Professor Brekhman showed mice given ginseng were able to swim nearly twice as long before they were exhausted.

The same experiment has been repeated in many parts of the world, with the same result. A European laboratory has recently demonstrated that even if the mice are given doses of ginseng which are the equivalent of normal human doses, their increase in stamina is still quite noticeable. The ginseng effect is cumulative.

If mice are given ginseng continuously for a month they can then regularly swim for twice as long as those mice not given ginseng.

The importance of these mice marathons lies in the fact that mice are not swimming longer because someone has told them how the Chinese Emperors enjoyed their ginseng, or because they saw a ginseng advert in the newspaper. The mice experiments show objectively that ginseng works, and its effects are not merely psychological. The studies also indicate that ginseng can be strong, especially in extreme situations. But they do not tell us very much about what ginseng is doing. Similar research has shown that caffeine, concentrated extracts of certain other plants such as basil, and even conventional anti-depressant drugs will increase the energy of mice in such stamina tests. Also the tests are not specially accurate nor are they particularly desirable from the animals' point of view.

Studies on people can give us more direct information, though in scientific terms they are less objective. The ginseng plant's effects were, traditionally, first discovered by the sensitive self-observation of herbalist — sages typified by the Emperor Shen Nung. The elaboration and understanding of how and when to take it for best results has come to us through millenia of careful observation. Science carries this a stage further. As an engineer will assess the strength of a structure by testing it under an excessive load, so human studies attempt to reveal the effects of ginseng by testing at extremes of stress or exhaustion.

Russian scientists have examined the effect of ginseng on human work capacity and energy by giving ginseng to proof readers, who are required to concentrate for longer than usual, and testing their speed and accuracy. Those given ginseng increased the number of letters read by twelve per cent and decreased the mistakes by fifty-one per cent compared with those given a 'mock extract' without ginseng. Similar results have been obtained when ginseng has been tested with people carrying out other demanding activities, such as high-speed radio telegraphy. It has been shown to improve the performance and capacity of students in a Swedish University undergoing tests, and of people doing exhausting physical work. In fact, the first study that convinced Soviet scientists that there was something in ginseng, and thus led to its verification in the laboratories of the world, involved 100 Soviet soldiers on a cross-country run. Those taking ginseng lopped some six per cent from their times, compared to the others taking a similar preparation without ginseng in it.

I have carried out a study at the Maudsley hospital, along with other doctors there, which tests ginseng under a very special condition of stress and tiredness: that of the switch-over from day work to night work. Nurses were given either Korean ginseng or a look-alike inert tablet for the first three days of their switch. After the third night, which is the one that they usually feel the most, they were all tested as to performance, energy, tiredness, ability to sleep during the day, and so on. It turned out that as expected, after switching to night work the nurses showed a considerable drop in alertness, energy, proficiency, activity and ability to work, and they felt poorly. Ginseng restored their performance (more than the inert look-alike) and mood, not all the way back to what it was during normal daytime working, but about half the way there. Though the nurses didn't sleep as well during the day, presumably because of the stimulation of the ginseng, they coped much better at night. This is after only three days at a small daily dose of just over 1 g of good quality Korean ginseng, equivalent to that recommended on the labels of most ginseng products in the shops.

Reflexes Speed up

Ginseng stimulates the nervous system itself. Reflexes have been shown to speed up; for example, tests have shown that the eye takes less time to adjust to the dark after taking ginseng. Professor Petkov, of the Institute of Advanced Medical Training in Sofia, has been occupied for the last fifteen years with elaborate experiments to assess its effects on the nervous system. He finds a typical stimulation of the brain wave patterns (electro-encephalogram) when experimental animals are given ginseng, and has repeatedly observed that the speed of conditioned (learned) behaviour in both animals and human subjects is increased. This implies an increase in efficiency of cerebral activity.

Professor Petkov has also shown the surprising phenomenon that mice which have learned a certain repetitive behaviour pattern, and then been allowed to forget it, could remember their training after a single low dose of ginseng corresponding to less than 1g for a human. Rats also showed an increased mental adaptability, since they could more easily switch from one type of learned response to another when given ginseng. He concluded from these types of experiment that: 'Ginseng stimulates . . . the basic neural processes which constitute the functioning of the cerebral cortex, namely the excitation . . . and inhibition . . . which form the physiological basis of man's mental functioning as a whole.' He continued, 'Ginseng, in contrast to other stimulants, causes no disturbance in the equilibrium of the cerebral processes. This explains the absence of any pronounced state of subjective excitement as is characteristic of all other stimulants . . . and also why this stimulant does not interfere with the normal course of sleep.'

Petkov felt that he had discovered a properly balanced stimulant, that is, a stimulant which actually improved the overall function of the mind and brain without paying for it with jittery over-arousal or subsequent exhaustion. To these scientists ginseng seemed to herald an utterly new generation of drug materials which, in some unknown way, could help man to cope more easily with the loads he carries. 'After various kinds of experiments on men,' writes Professor Petkov, 'it was established that daily doses of ginseng preparations during 15-45 days increase physical endurance and mental capacity for work, as well as industrial activity.' The increase in work efficiency was noted not only during the treatment itself but also for a stated period of time (a month and a half) after the treatment was over.

Japanese researchers have studied how ginseng stimulates by simply watching and measuring the activity of animals who had been given ginseng extract compared to others given a similar but dummy liquid. The animals given ginseng showed more general activity. They explored their environment — running up nets and through holes — more frequently than their colleagues. The difference was especially pronounced when the animals were tired from previous exercise.

In keeping with its action on the nervous system, ginseng has been shown to reverse and block the effects of alcohol and sedative drugs such as barbiturates and chlorpromazine. Yet, strangely, it has been demonstrated that there is a sedative component in the root itself. Japanese scientists at the University of Tokyo showed that rats given very high doses of ginseng extract in addition to a sleeping draught slept more and were less restless than with the sleeping draught alone.

How is it possible, one might ask at this point, for a drug to have both a stimulating and a sedative effect? It is indeed possible, and there need be no paradox. It has been shown that ginseng contains a number of components, some of which can work in opposite ways. Japanese scientists, particularly, have carried out extensive and highly sophisticated tests of behaviour and activity in animals. They find that certain components increase activity and learning ability, and others decrease it. This is one plausible explanation for the balanced action noticed by Petkov; that alertness is increased but the ability to rest, relax and sleep is also preserved.

A remedy that can have apparently opposite effects is no mystery in the herbal tradition. Indeed, such remedies are treasured, for the value of a single preparation that can pick you up if you are over-tired, yet will prevent you from becoming over-excited, is obvious.

——Ginseng Compared with Other Stimulants——

As both Professor Petkov and Professor Brekhman have remarked in their reports, there is a world of difference between ginseng and other stimulants such as caffeine or amphetamine.

(a) Ginseng is not an excitant. It does not cause feelings of over-excitation, emotional disturbance or agitation in humans, nor, as far as can be judged, in animals.

(b) There is a sedative component in ginseng. Unlike other stimulants, there is no difficulty in sleeping after taking it.

(c) Ginseng acts in a stabilizing fashion. The more tired one is, the more noticeable is its action.

(d) Ginseng causes an increase in health, appetite and mental condition, especially if taken over a period. The other stimulants cause more ill health the longer they are taken.

(e) Ginseng is much safer than other stimulants.

(f) Ginseng may assist in combating stress, while the other stimulants can actually cause stress.

─────────────**Ginseng and Stress**─────────────

The body has automatic mechanisms which are called upon if a dangerous or potentially harmful situation arises. Loud noises, threats, wounding, the potential of a wound, fear, anger, emotional tension and so on, all generate the automatic stress response. The response is controlled by hormones. Hormones are chemical substances made in various glands around the body which control and integrate the body metabolism and co-ordinate the response of the body to the world outside. They are like nerves, but their message is slower; if nerves are the body's telephone system, then hormones would be the postal service. The stress response is governed by hormones secreted from the adrenal glands, just above the kidneys. These hormones produce a state of readiness and mobilization in the body. Blood is shifted away from 'peacetime' functions, such as digestion, to the muscles. The heart speeds up, blood vessels contract, blood pressure rises, the metabolism changes, the pattern of the body defences against injury and infection alters and the mind becomes aroused.

While occasional stress is often necessary and can help to keep one alert and motivated, too much stress is undoubtedly bad for the body. Whether it is stress from outside, such as experienced by busy administrators or workers in a noisy factory, or from inside, in tense and anxious people, continuous stress is disastrous for health. It lowers resistance to disease, contributes to high blood-pressure and cardiovascular problems, has been implicated in cancer, and is a direct cause of digestive troubles, gastric ulcer, tiredness, insomnia, migraines and other diseases. The body is drained of vitality when its defences are overworked.

In a study that I carried out with other scientists at Chelsea College, University of London, we tested an idea about ginseng first put forward by Professor Brekhman. That is, that it helps one overcome stress and challenge. We gave ginseng extract to many mice while a similar number had the inevitable pretend extract. We watched the general behaviour of the mice. Then we put the mice in a situation of mild stress. We placed them on a large white disc under a light, a situation they find somewhat alarming, accustomed as they are to corners and dark holes.

It turned out that the mice which had the ginseng could hardly be distinguished from the others during their normal periods of activity. However as soon as they were placed under stress their reactions were much more pronounced. They explored, crouched and went into their alert defensive rituals a great deal more than those not given ginseng.

The major success of scientific research on ginseng is that it has repeatedly been shown that ginseng helps the body to cope with stress. In laboratories in Korea, Russia, Bulgaria, America and London, mice under stress have been given ginseng. They showed two basic improvements. Firstly, there was an increase in the weight and function of the adrenal glands, together with less abnormalities of behaviour and distress: the mice were, in fact, more able to 'absorb' stress. One is reminded of the Chinese soldiers who take ginseng with them to the battlefield to help them resist the effects of stress and shock. Secondly, there was an actual *reduction* in the long-term stress response and its corresponding harmful effects. The body had increased its resistance. When ginseng was taken, the animals coped better with actual stress but the body activity settled back to normal more quickly. It is now felt that this is a key to ginseng's reputed ability to increase health.

An Adaptogen?

A consideration of the way ginseng can cause resistance to stress leads inevitably to one of the most exciting ideas in pharmacology. Professor Brekhman, and also scientists in South Korea, carried out the following experiments. Mice were given ginseng and subjected to the depressant action of chloral hydrate, barbiturates and alcohol; and their recovery improved. They were irradiated with X-rays, the most damaging of influences on the body, and their resistance doubled. The mice also showed a greater ability to survive after being given a fiendish collection of poisons and drugs such as potent anti-cancer drugs, after infection with bacteria, and after stress by physical conditions such as heat, cold and change in pressure.

Chemical changes in the body were then measured to see how the mice were coping. The surprising fact is that ginseng had no effect on these processes in the absence of stress. In other words, it only acted to return the body to normal if it had gone off course. This has led to the exciting concept of using the plant as an 'adaptogen' — a medicine which increases the ability of the body to adapt, and which only works when it is needed. The idea is unique in Western drug research and, apart from ginseng and its relatives within oriental medicine, no other drug or medicine is known which has a 'normalizing' effect. To most scientists who have been studying the action of drugs, it would seem hard to believe that such a thing exists. But the evidence is plain for everyone to see and is published in the scientific literature. The Chinese, of course, have recognized this property of ginseng for a long time. They have always stated that ginseng adjusts or harmonizes body functions that have gone astray. They are justified in saying, 'I told you so'. A harmless medicine which returns wayward body processes to normal, however mild the effect, may be described as an ideal medicine. The medicine of the past may well turn out to be a medicine of the future.

How can ginseng work as an adaptogen? It is difficult to know exactly, because it has so many different effects on the body. The secret is likely to be in the way that it acts on the hormones. If ginseng improves the efficiency of the hormone messenger systems, then one might expect a greater co-ordination in the defence forces of the body. The body is helped to help itself, whether the problem is abnormal blood-pressure or abnormal tiredness.

There is evidence that ginseng does indeed stimulate several glands to regulate their hormone production. Korean and Chinese research has shown that ginseng does act directly on the adrenal glands, although there are other studies that show that resistance is improved, even when the adrenal glands are removed. We can suggest that some of the actions of ginseng are through the adrenal glands, while others, as Professor Petkov has shown, may be on the brain itself.

Alertness and Challenge

There is an interesting connection between the way ginseng improves alertness and well-being, and the way it protects against stress and strain. Common sense tells us that there is a natural linkage between mental wakefulness and the stress response. For example challenge — things that go bump in the night, or the starting line of an athletic event — is a considerable stimulant to the brain. Too much challenge — continuous anxiety, executive stress, or long hours on the production line — saps the available mental energy leading to exhaustion and that feeling of being drained. Scientists know how challenge wakes up the mind. It does so initially through the production of adrenaline. At the same time, the stress hormones, called corticosteroids, that as we have seen are released by the adrenal glands, travel to the brain and produce motivation, alertness and a readiness to act just as they travel to the muscles and circulation and alert them too.

There is evidence that ginseng facilitates this linkage between mind and body. For a start the kind of wakefulness produced by ginseng is very similar to that produced by these corticosteroids. It is an increased alertness, motivation, energy and even well-being, which is also experienced by patients who have received such hormones for medical conditions. Experiments in which tired animals have had to work out how to negotiate mazes, or tired people have had to solve problems or transmit in morse code, show too that ginseng creates a mental readiness and capacity just as if challenged. It is completely different from the speediness produced by all known stimulants which act by accelerating mental activity.

In studies carried out by Dr Deepak Shori and myself at the University of London it became clear that ginseng increased the amount of these corticosteroid hormones getting to the brain, for after giving animals a measured amount of these hormones, much more was found located in the brain of those animals given ginseng than those which had been given a dummy preparation. Dr Hiai and other scientists at Toyama University, Toyama, in Japan, have gone even further. In a long investigation covering years of work they have shown that ginseng acts on the regulation systems in the brain, located in the glands called the hypothalamus and pituitary, that actually direct the state of readiness in both the body and the mind. It is these glands which receive messages from the senses calling for mobilization, and then tell the adrenal glands to send out their stress hormones.

In other words, improved stamina and alertness, and resistance to stress, are actually the same thing, brought on by more efficient physiological co-ordination. Ginseng makes a little hormone go a long way.

Tuning and Toning

The Soviet researchers describe ginseng as an adaptogen. The research we have carried out shows how ginseng helps to harmonize our mind and body. These are modern descriptions corresponding exactly to the claims of the ancient Chinese. Their 'adjustive', 'kingly' remedy we know to be adaptogenic, or regulatory, their 'yang' we know to be alerting, arousing, awakening. It is as if ginseng tunes our engines to make them work more efficiently. We get a higher performance with less fuel. Interestingly, 'tuning' and 'toning' come from the same word. Ginseng conforms to the original meaning of the word 'tonic', an agent which adjusts the body and mind to make it function better.

This plant is not alone in this category. Many other 'kingly' Chinese plants make parts of the body function more efficiently: for example liquorice acts on the water balance in the body through other hormones; pantocrine, or deer horn, appears to help in the sexual or generative area; *Bupleurum* improves liver function; *Schizandra chinensis* tunes the carbohydrate metabolism; *Angelica chinensis* treats disturbances in female hormones and restores poor vitality especially in women. All of these kingly remedies have the interesting property of having very little effect when the body/mind are in good condition, well-motivated, well-functioning, vital and energetic. They only tend to work when the system is thrown out of balance.

CHAPTER 5

Mincing the Man Root

A plant with such subtle properties has provided chemists with an irresistible temptation to take it to bits and to try and find out which substances are responsible. Until the early 1960s all that was detected in the root was the usual carbohydrates, cellulose, minerals and other common constituents that you would expect to find in a parsnip or a potato. However during the early 1960s, after it had been clearly demonstrated that ginseng could increase the stamina of mice, scientists began to take the root apart chemically, and see which agents were able to achieve the same results as the whole root. Professor Elyakov's team in Moscow University, and Professor Shibata's team in Tokyo began a race to find the key ingredients of ginseng, producing a flurry of reports much to the mystification of the rest of the scientific world at the time who couldn't understand what the fuss was about.

Using modern analytical techniques, they found that compounds called *terpenoidal glycosides* could give the mice as much extra stamina as if they had been given the whole root. These are somewhat soapy materials made up of sugar molecules connected to a terpenoid molecule — a plant hormone that looks quite like the human hormones we have been talking about. These glycosides are made in the leaves, flowers and peel of the root, and then transported down to be stored in the flesh of the root. There may be two to six per cent of these materials in the dry root. Sixteen different glycosides have now been identified and their chemical structure revealed. They have been named by the Japanese researchers *ginsenosides,* and coded Ra, Rb, Rc . . . etc. The proportion of the various ginsenosides varies according to the way the root is grown, which location it comes from, its age, variety, method of drying and so on. Thus American ginseng can be distinguished from Asian ginseng by having more ginsenosides of less variety, with Ra, Rf and Rh absent. The ginsenosides are maximum in August, just before harvest, and they increase with age.

Now that the main active materials are known, it is possible to set a standard, that is the requirement that all ginseng in the market must have a minimum amount of ginsenosides (usually one or two per cent) for it to be described as pure ginseng. This has happened in the United States and such a standard is also present in the 1987 Swiss Pharmacopoiea.

Many of the medicinal properties of ginseng root tested in the laboratory can be repeated using the ginsenosides alone. They have been shown to be stimulatory, to reduce stress, increase stamina, wakefulness and performance, to affect the adrenal glands and the hormones, to increase the metabolism in the liver and other organs, to affect the circulation, etc. Some interesting discoveries have emerged, for example that Re and Rg are more stimulatory and Rc and Rb are more sedative. Therefore differences in the amounts of each type could explain how some roots, for example American ginseng, are more yin or quietening, while others, for example Korean red ginseng, are more yang or arousing.

However, the situation is not yet clear. For it turns out that in some good quality roots, such as six year red ginseng, there will be less ginsenoside than in poor quality ginseng, such as four year old pencil roots. Besides, root hairs and tendrils are of poor quality and less effect, even though their ginsenoside levels are extremely high. In fact the Koreans traditionally throw away a lot of the ginsenosides in the peel when they peel roots for steaming. Add to this the fact that infected or damaged roots have increased ginsenosides, and it will be clear that one cannot make the equation that ginsenosides = medicinal effects. It has been suggested, as a way out of this problem, that it is not the actual amounts of ginsenosides in the roots that gives the effects, but their quantities relative to each other. This may be true but is as yet unproven.

It is more likely that there are other compounds unrelated to the ginsenosides that are contributing to ginseng's effects. A few are becoming known, most are still unknown. For example a small protein material has been found in ginseng which seems to be responsible for helping sugar and fat metabolism. A group of compounds termed plant phenols, in particular a compound called maltol, have been found to help in protection of the tissues and possibly in reducing some of the damage due to ageing. We also know that ginseng contains essential oils, fats, ginsenin, phytosterin, resins, mucilaginous compounds, vitamins, sugars, certain alkaloids, minerals, silicic acids, and other compounds. It is clear that there are many compounds in ginseng which add up to the total effect of the root. Ginseng is a good example of a herb in which it is proven that the whole is greater than the sum of its parts.

A question that might be raised is whether the ginsenosides, or terpenoidal glycosides in general, appear in other plants and if so, whether they have ginseng-like properties. The ginsenosides are unique and are found only in ginseng, and its relatives. However there are terpenoidal glycosides in many plants, especially those with medicinal properties recognized by Chinese medicine. The kingly remedies have them; as do plants such as liquorice, the jujube, *Bupleurum* species, *Platycodon* species, *Polygala* species (such as snakeroot), or *Schizandra*. While in western medicine the sedative *Valerian* and the tonics *Sarsaparilla* and *Spikenard* are among the well-known plants in which triterpenoid glycosides could be the active ingredients. In all cases they have mild, tonic, adjustive actions. It is this mildness which has prevented western scientists from taking the triterpenoid glycosides seriously. You won't find them in textbooks of pharmacology. Conventional research into drugs is looking for strong curative chemicals, not mild, adjustive or preventive ones.

CHAPTER 6

—Ginseng and Disease—

Ginseng does not cure any specific disease or any specific symptom. However it can improve the state of health, of vitality, of adaptability or resistance, and this may prevent a disease or nip it in the bud. In particular, ginseng may aid in a number of diseases which are endemic to the modern world and are the result of too much stress and strain. Some ten per cent of the population of America suffers from high blood pressure or other circulatory problems upon which there is known to be a strong influence of anxiety, stress and tension. Cancer risk is increased by grief or despair, and in laboratory studies with animals, by stress or crowding. Even infections are more easily caught when you are in difficult circumstances. The way stress creates holes in our immunity is becoming much clearer today; it is a science with its own name — psychoneuroimmunology. The hormones we have been discussing above are very much involved in the weakening of the immunity by unremitting stress.

Ginseng might be expected to reduce the damage created by excessive stress for it tightens up the physiological systems that react to it. The result should be improved immunity, resistance to infections and possibly even cancer, and a reduction in circulatory and other diseases that arise from inner imbalance. We will examine these in turn.

Preventing Infections

During 1975-1980 no less than 60,000 Soviet car workers at the Volzhsky car factory in Togliatti were given a daily dose of extract of eleutherococcus for several months. Their general health improved, the number of days off work was substantially reduced, and they seemed to be in better cardiovascular condition than the rest of the workers. This kind of study has been carried out with several kinds of Soviet workers, especially long distance lorry drivers, albeit with ginseng relatives rather than ginseng itself. The Russians have stated that their aim is to reduce ill-health among workers vulnerable because of industrial stress. They appear to have succeeded, and both ginseng and eleutherococcus are now available in the USSR for this purpose. Similar observations have been reported from European old peoples' homes, where old people given ginseng appear to be rather more healthy, active and resistant to disease. On the other hand it is difficult to prove that it was the ginseng that benefited the patients, or other salutary influences, and the same criticism can be levelled at the Soviet trials, however massive.

Nevertheless there is some scientific support for the traditional claim that doses of ginseng at the right time can help to restore weakened resistance. Animals given ginseng and then infected with disease-causing bacteria are less likely to be ill. In Japan, researchers have found that ginseng can perk up the immune system — both the white cells that stand guard and the antibodies that are their weapons. Ginseng is known to enrich the blood with protective cells and their manufacture in the bone marrow noticeably speeds up. There is even research from the Central Drug Research Laboratory in Lucknow, India, suggesting that members of the ginseng family may be able to stimulate the body to produce more interferon, the anti-viral protective protein that is much in the news these days.

It is important not to regard ginseng as some kind of plant antibiotic. It has no effect whatever against bacteria, viruses or other infectious agents. Instead it would help to shore up immunity that is reduced by exhaustion, strain or poor vitality. However, even in this role ginseng does not provide a quick fix. There are, in fact, many other oriental plants which have a stronger and more specific action on the immunity. Rather, it should be seen as part of a health maintenance programme, in the Chinese fashion, in which ginseng works alongside dietary control and a healthy lifestyle.

Ginseng and Cancer

In so far as cancer arises through depressed immunity, ginseng, especially when combined with healthy habits, may have a general preventive effect against cancer. The restoration of vitality and well-being will make cancer less likely. However ginseng does not have any effect on cancer itself, just as it has no effect on invading bacteria. There is one important potential use of ginseng in this disease, and that is as a support during cancer treatment. Modern treatment is stressful, debilitating and damaging to the immunity. Although it is able to destroy primary cancers, the patient is often left more vulnerable against secondaries. Studies on animals in the USSR by Dr Yaremenko and his colleagues have indicated that eleutherococcus can protect the body from the stress of surgery and drug treatment. Surgery was found to increase the chances of secondary growths through stress, while eleutherococcus prevented this increase. Korean scientists have reported similar findings using ginseng. Both eleutherococcus and ginseng have been shown to protect patients from some of the damage and debility caused by radiotherapy. The patients were better able to tolerate the treatment, with less side effects such as nausea and tiredness. At the famous Petrov Oncological Institute in Leningrad, it was found that one teaspoonful of concentrated eleutherococcus extract per day enabled patients to cope successfully with 50 per cent more anti-cancer drugs, and they lived longer as a result.

Ginseng and especially eleutherococcus are now used quite widely in the USSR for this purpose. There is also a range of specialized plant remedies in use in China to assist the health and immunity of the patient during medical treatment of cancer. This subject is discussed further in my recent book, *How To Survive Medical Treatment*. These materials have been in regular use in this manner for 20 years without western doctors taking any notice. This indicates, unfortunately, that conventional medicine is still concentrating on assaulting the disease, leaving the patient an unprotected battlefield.

Convalescence

Convalescence is a period of debility and reduced vitality in which ginseng can be very useful. This must not be confused with the cure of disease, for which ginseng cannot be used. Ginseng's role would begin when the battle against the disease has already been won, but the body still needs to recover its strength. This has been investigated in the case of tuberculosis by Soviet and Korean scientists, who find that ginseng and eleutherococcus have no effect in the acute phase of the disease, but shorten the recovery stage. A recent study in a Korean hospital has clearly demonstrated that ginseng's glycosides can aid recovery of patients who have had serious operations.

─────────────Ginseng and Circulation─────────────

Studies have also shown that ginseng may be of assistance in the all-too-common disease of the circulation. When ginseng was given to dogs with artificially raised blood pressure, the blood pressure was somewhat lowered. Likewise, animals with sharply reduced blood pressure showed a significant return to normality. In clinical trials with elderly patients who had high blood pressure, ginseng was shown to produce a consistent but small reduction in the blood pressure.

Ginseng, being a yang or heating remedy, tends to raise (or 'heat up') lowered blood pressure more quickly and easily than it lowers raised blood pressure. After a number of clinical studies in Chinese hospitals, the Chinese now use ginseng as part of emergency treatment to restore blood pressure and keep the patient going after shock (i.e. loss of blood) and heart attacks. It appears to be more effective, especially when in combination with other herbs, than any known conventional drug used for this purpose.

At the same time, Soviet and German doctors report that ginseng will help to reduce high blood pressure, but it must be used as part of a global nature-cure treatment that includes diet or fasting, exercise and relaxation. Ginseng would in this case help the body to adjust to its new lifestyle, burn up waste products and stabilize the metabolism. There are several studies suggesting that ginseng reduces cholesterol in the circulation. This is not a primary action — it is not a specific cholesterol-lowering agent — but it is secondary to re-adjustment to a more active, cleaner metabolism. Interestingly, because American ginseng is more yin, and less arousing, it may be more successful in this regard than Asian ginseng. According to Dr Elson at the University of

Wisconsin, American ginseng is most successful at lowering cholesterol levels in animal experiments.

The way that ginseng can both lower and raise blood pressure may seem a puzzle to some. However the puzzle is not created by ginseng. It is rather the result of western assumptions that a drug ought to change some body process in one direction only. In fact in oriental medicine remedies that work in more than one direction are the norm. For the action of adjustive medicines depend on the background — they act as they are needed — raising, lowering or doing nothing according to the state of the patient.

Energy and Metabolism

Diabetes is a disturbance of the metabolism of sugar in the liver. Administration of ginseng to animals tends to reduce the blood sugar, in those with artificially raised blood sugar. This stabilizing effect is a typical adaptogenic one, since ginseng has also been shown to *raise* blood sugar when it is artificially lowered by insulin injections. It can aid but not replace medical treatment. In China, ginseng and other herbs may be given to people with diabetes not as a replacement for insulin or injections, but as a way of helping their body adjust to the injected insulin. Acupuncture has a similar role to play in Chinese medicine, which it may do more successfully than ginseng by itself. It is used to help allay some of the potential damage that may be done to the tissues of diabetics despite the insulin.

Ginseng has a subtle effect on many different types of metabolism, and research is being carried on at the moment in order to try to understand its action on the chemical processes in the body. Dr Aviakian, of the University of California, and his colleagues have recently discovered, for example, that it causes more economical use of body-energy and an extra storage of energy-producing compounds in the liver. If animals are forced to take extensive exercise, the supply of energy is not so depleted in the presence of ginseng. It has also been discovered that ginseng can regulate the basal metabolic rate, often raising it when it is too slow, to increase the breakdown and metabolism of foods, liberating more energy and removing more waste products. These kinds of metabolic effects may be responsible for the suggestions that ginseng can prevent hangovers. Certainly the Russians think so and encourage people to take eleutherococcus or ginseng with or after their vodka, and an eleutherococcus-vodka is on sale there. Ginseng also increases the rate of 'manufacture' of important body chemicals in the liver. It is not certain if these are direct effects of ginseng or the secondary result of the stimulation of the hormone system. Interestingly, ginseng can stimulate the metabolism of body cells even when the cells are isolated and kept in a test tube, so hormones are not always needed for it to work.

Ginseng and Potency

One of the many fabled powers of ginseng is that it increases sexual vitality. Science has something to say about this, namely that ginseng cannot stimulate sexual performance, except in a psychological or suggestive manner. Therefore if it is believed that it increases sexual prowess, then it probably will, because sexual virility is to some extent a matter of confidence.

Many drugs and medicines have been hopefully called 'aphrodisiacs', but there are in fact very few real aphrodisiacs and it is doubtful if ginseng is one of them. On the other hand, there is scientific evidence that it may have the less dramatic but nevertheless important function of helping to restore male potency in some cases of impotence. Many cases of impotence are psychological, but some are due to a decline in the hormones which control the sexual responses. There is clear evidence that ginseng contains compounds with sex hormone activity, and in some experiments it has been shown to reverse harmful effects due to a lack of male sex hormones.

In other experiments the ginseng glycosides were able to encourage the development of the sex organs in young animals. Young mice given ginseng reached puberty faster than untreated mice, and they had prostate glands forty to sixty per cent larger. In fact, the increase in weight of these glands has been suggested by Professor Brekhman as a way of measuring the strength of different ginseng preparations. Dr Karzel of the University of Bonn concludes: 'The occurrence of constituents with sex-hormone-like activity in ginseng preparations thus seems to be proven . . . but questions concerning the ratios between male and female hormones remain to be solved.'

There are clinical reports from Russia of striking improvements when ginseng was given to some patients suffering from sexual impotence. The patients felt more tranquil and active, and showed an improvement in sexual function. Although much more study is needed, we can say that perhaps the Chinese are justified in expecting to be fertile in old age with the help of ginseng.

CHAPTER 7

————The Elixir?————

The Chinese have always been interested in old age. While European alchemists were devoted to the attempt to convert dross into gold, the Chinese alchemists were similarly occupied with finding the elixir of life. The herbal manuals are insistent that ginseng can prolong life, although they recognize that it certainly is not 'The Elixir': 'If even the herb Chu-seng can make one live longer, try putting the Elixir in the mouth' says an alchemist book of AD 142.

Of all the people who treasure ginseng in China, it is the old who are most enthusiastic. As we have seen, the common belief is that if taken regularly, it will retard the ageing process, keeping crippling diseases such as arthritis and cardiovascular disease at bay, provide energy to old people with flagging vitality, and would even allow men to retain their sexual potency until the very last years of their life. The very best gift an old man or woman could receive in China would be a good ginseng root.

Much of the lore and ritual concerning the use of ginseng is perpetuated by the elderly. They are the ones who keep ginseng soaking in brandy for years, waiting for the most auspicious occasion to consume it; who respect ginseng for its supposed radiation and keep it in lead-lined boxes; who will spend their life's savings on select roots. Mao Tse-Tung and Chou en-Lai were both known to take ginseng regularly. Father Jartoux was also in complete agreement with the Chinese belief that ginseng was able to prolong life and wrote enthusiastically about it.

————The Ageing Process————
Can ginseng really help a man to resist the effects of ageing? This

is really two questions. Is such a thing as a 'Fountain of Youth' possible? If so, would ginseng qualify as one? In order to answer these questions we have to know something more about the ageing process.

Ageing is inevitable. Despite the biblical statement that Methusaleh and others lived many hundreds of years, it is accepted that the potential lifespan is limited to about 110 years. Well before this time the body begins to run down. The correct workings of the organs, cells, the bodily metabolism slowly deteriorate. Scientists have recently demonstrated that the very information which controls the construction and smooth running of the body wears itself out, just like the message on a tape will become obscured after many re-runs through a tape recorder. This is the *process* of ageing.

The *effects* of ageing are visible deteriorations that arise from this process. As ageing continues, the body becomes more and more vulnerable to disease and damage. Old people are increasingly likely to catch infections, for example, or they tend to have slower reactions and are therefore more likely to be involved in a road accident.

Resisting the Effects of Ageing

The *process* of ageing cannot be altered or manipulated by any external agent. Scientists admit that a real elixir of life is not foreseeable. Immortality is a myth and it will remain so. This is not so gloomy as it sounds, because the *effects* of ageing can be mollified. The motto of the American Gerontological Society is 'To Add Life to Years not Years to Life'.

Supposing it were possible so to increase the resistance of the body that despite ageing continuing at its own pace, no premature illnesses were suffered by the old person. In that case the person would reach his potential lifespan. He would be healthy and active until the day he died. He would just 'die of old age' when his body could not function any more. Country people in some Shangri-La areas of the world — secluded valleys in the mountains of South Russia, Hunza in Pakistan, Vilcabambas in Ecuador — have a number of very old people who are healthy and are reaching their maximum potential lifespan. It may be 100 years or just over.

In general, any treatment that improves the health and fitness of the body can be expected to assist in resisting the effects of ageing, despite the ageing process itself continuing at the same rate. Yoga and exercise can both have an effect on the lifespan in this way. Alternatively, cigarette smoking can shorten the lifespan by making the body more vulnerable to cancer and bronchial infections.

Every culture has traditional remedies and treatments which are purported to lead to a healthy long life. In the West a proliferation of possible substances has been in the news, such as vitamin C, vitamin E, unsaturated oils in food, procaine, anti-oxidants (similar to food preservatives) and synthetic hormones. In addition, comfrey root, liquorice, garlic and vegetarian food are traditional suggestions.

In India there is a special section of traditional medicine, called *Rasaaynen,* which is devoted to resisting the effects of ageing. This treatment is of great antiquity and complexity. It involves an elaborate series of herbs which are to be taken over a long period while the subject is living inside a specially built room or cell, the precise measurements of which are laid down. Some noted Indian politicians, such as Jawaharlal Nehru, are known to have undergone this process.

The Chinese, of course, have a rich source of different herbal medicines which are useful in combating ageing symptoms, but none of the same repute as ginseng. One Peking professor, reported the *New York Times* in 1933, lived for 256 years. This should not be taken too seriously, but it is of interest that he attributed his purported longevity to a tea that he brewed daily. The tea contained ginseng and 'Fo ti teng', which is either *Hydrocotyle asiatica,* a common creeping plant, or the Chinese medicine *Polygonum multiflora.*

In the early twenties, Claude Bernard, a distinguished scientist, introduced a fashion for eating the gonads of monkeys as a way of prolonging life. Scientists at that time believed that ageing was due to the failure of the hormones of the body and that taking hormones in this form could slow down the process.

A rather less crude development of hormone therapy arrived with the availability of synthetic hormones such as testosterone. Testosterone is still taken nowadays, although only in special cases of premature impotence or decline in virility. It has certain harmful side effects with prolonged use.

In theory, hormone therapy could slow down some of the effects of ageing, because the efficiency of the internal hormones does indeed decline with age. Taking hormones will compensate, but only for a limited period.

Ginseng and Ageing

The Chinese find European involvement with monkey glands amusing. Why, they ask, does one need to eat monkey glands when a natural plant exists which is much more effective, longer lasting and safer? The intriguing fact is that ginseng also seems to act very much as a hormone, but in addition stimulates the body to produce its own hormones. This may be one way in which it could moderate the effects of ageing.

We have also seen how a decline in resistance is a key manifestation of ageing. Ginseng is almost the only known substance which can increase bodily resistance. One of the major effects of ageing, especially in the developed countries, is a degeneration of the blood system causing strokes, heart attacks, etc. We know that ginseng helps to treat cardiovascular diseases and diabetes. Another complaint of the elderly is tiredness, and we have demonstrated that ginseng is a safe and effective long term stimulant. All these factors would suggest that ginseng is ideal for treatment of the symptoms of ageing.

There is unfortunately very little scientific evidence on this aspect of ginseng. It would be difficult to demonstrate an effect on the lifespan of humans, because it would take so long that the scientists would be old at the end of the experiment.

Animals can be used, however; the lifespan of a mouse is two years. Observations on the effect of ginseng on the lifespan of mice have been carried out by myself and others at the University of London. Mice were given very small doses of ginseng throughout their life. The treated mice appeared more active and there were fewer deaths in that group for some time after ginseng was given, compared to a similar group of mice that were not given ginseng. However, the lifespan was not altered to any major extent. Soviet scientists have reported that a colony of rats given ginseng lived considerably longer than a similar colony without, but this awaits confirmation.

It is also possible to carry out experiments on human cells isolated from the body. Ginseng has been shown by myself and other scientists to stimulate the growth of such cells, and to delay the death and disintegration of the cells under inhospitable conditions. Such experiments are just the beginning.

────────Tests Just Beginning────────

Trials of ginseng with old people in hospitals and old-age homes are also getting off the ground. They have already given encouraging results. In one case, sixty-six patients in the age range thirty to sixty were given ginseng and vitamins. Improvements were noticed in most of the patients who suffered from cardiovascular diseases, depression and reduced vitality. There were also psychological benefits. Many of the patients revealed an awakening of interest in life. The psychological aspects are also the most marked feature of another recent clinical trial. Two German doctors gave ginseng to ninety-five patients in old-age homes. Besides improvements in blood pressure, memory, neurological function and bodily function, fifty-eight of the patients showed 'an enhancement of mood so marked as to be almost euphoric, and in almost all cases it was maintained for a period of months'. The doctors then continue: 'It goes without saying that tiredness or exhaustion was one of our patients main symptoms . . . 83 per cent showed clear improvements in both these syndromes, which can be considered an excellent result.'

Another study has been in progress for some time in East Germany under supervision of the top gerontologists there. Almost 600 people are being examined. First results indicate that ginseng does improve their well-being.

Dr Kataria, a consultant gerontologist of St Francis's hospital in London, together with myself and a nurse, Beryl Gethyn-Smith, have recently studied the effects of good quality Korean red ginseng root in a 'double-blind' study on 60 old people who complained of tiredness and of being run down. They took the ginseng for 10 days, and on another occasion took a look-alike preparation for 10 days. Neither the old people nor the nurse who saw them knew which was which. We found that when they took ginseng there was a very clear improvement in their alertness, speed of reaction, and co-ordination at tasks which we set for them. However they didn't seem to notice any change in themselves for they did not record that they felt any better.

It may be true to say that ginseng is ideal for old people. It is my belief that the Chinese have introduced to the world the only drug or medicine which has ever been shown to have medicinal powers which specifically fit the conditions of the elderly. Others who have researched into ginseng also hold this view. Professor Brekhman has been claiming for many years that ginseng would be of great interest to gerontologists (those studying ageing). One international company has been marketing a geriatric preparation for some time which is widely available in Europe. Its main constituent is ginseng.

Not an Elixir

A note of caution is necessary. It can be dangerous to raise false hopes. We have shown that ginseng cannot be regarded as an elixir. It can only palliate the effects of ageing. Even this it does in a mild and gentle manner, building up over a long period. Like many other herbs, it works gradually and the effects are not violent and dramatic. Moreover, it cannot be expected to cure the degenerative diseases of old age. It is likely to produce a mild improvement, but its main function would be to help the body resist developing these conditions in the first place. For this purpose it must be taken continuously and regularly. It is well known that people vary considerably in their response to drugs and herbs and the effects of ginseng may or may not be immediately noticeable depending on other factors such as diet, the quality of the root and so on.

There are other ways in which old people could maximize the chances of attaining a healthy old age, which are probably in the long run more effective than any tonics, including ginseng. Diet should be moderate, with plenty of roughage, fresh fruit and vegetables or grains, avoiding fatty and rich foods, sugar and starch. Exercise should be regular and sufficiently vigorous, and should be maintained throughout life because it is difficult and even dangerous to begin vigorous exercise in advanced age. Stress-free living, a sanguine and calm existence, is essential to health. This includes an intelligent avoidance of harmful environmental influences.

CHAPTER 8

How to Take Ginseng

Both the claims made for ginseng by the Chinese and the experiments of modern science can be used for a practical purpose: to inform those who are interested in taking ginseng how to take it. The following are the uses for which ginseng can be recommended.

(a) *Stimulant.* Ginseng has been shown to be a safe, effective and natural stimulant with many advantages over other stimulants such as caffeine or amphetamines. It can be taken for tiredness and exhaustion, or when going through a heavily taxing task, such as examinations, long-distance driving, stage performances, unusually strenuous physical work and so on. It is ideally suited for those occasions when one is exhausted from overwork, insomnia or over-indulgence, and may be a very effective way of coping with a hangover. In these cases it should be taken at the time when it is needed. The doses are given on page 69.

(b) *Tonic.* The Chinese tend to pay more attention to ginseng as a long-term restorative, because it is believed that benefits to health only accrue from the gradual and continuous use of natural medicines. It is recommended in convalescence from disease, in coping with long-term tiredness, or in removing the feeling of being below par ('one degree under'). Taking ginseng at these times may not only remove the feeling of being off colour and tired, but also decrease the likelihood of incurring a disease due to lowered bodily resistance. It may also be taken for diseases such as anaemia and dysentry, where tiredness is a side effect.

(c) *Mental benefits.* Judging from the Russian experience with ginseng for improving the mental state of the elderly, there are also psychological benefits to be obtained from its long-term use.

It can be recommended for depression and insomnia, as it has been documented repeatedly that it is able to raise spirits and improve outlook on life, especially among the elderly. Its general tonic effects may also assist memory and concentration.

(d) *Anti-stress.* Ginseng taken regularly may assist in coping with the stress and strains of life. It may also help the body resist the harmful long-term effect of stress which, as we have seen, can produce a general deterioration of health and well-being.

(e) *Regulating blood pressure.* Although it has been demonstrated to have a mild stabilizing effect on blood pressure, whether low or high, the causes of irregular blood pressure are often inherent changes in the cardiovascular system, and they cannot actually be reversed or cured by ginseng. It can safely be taken as a regular course by those with disorders of the cardiovascular system, but it should be on a trial and error basis, and with the full knowledge and consent of the individual's doctor. Ginseng can normally be taken in addition to any other drugs which may have been prescribed.

(f) *Anti-diabetic.* As there is some evidence that ginseng can adjust the blood sugar level in cases of diabetes, it may be taken by diabetics along with other treatment, and if there is a noticeable improvement this can be taken into account in the long-term management of the disease. Again, there will be no problems of incompatibility with other treatments as the herb is mild and extremely safe. It is better to be dependent on ginseng to assist in the management of a particular disease — if it helps — than to be dependent on stronger allopathic medicines.

(g) *Against impotence.* This is an area of treatment full of 'quackery' and old wives' tales. As we have seen, impotence may be psychological rather more often than physical, and ginseng may help certain cases of physical impotence, particularly where it is the result of a general lack of vitality. Chinese doctors have placed great faith in long-term courses of ginseng for the treatment of physical impotence, and especially the decline in potency which accompanies ageing. Incidentally, the Chinese say that when it is used for the treatment of flagging vitality (both sexual and otherwise), it should be accompanied by a period of continence. They believe that continence will cause secretions which arise through the use of ginseng to become reabsorbed into the blood stream and thus revitalize the brain and body. The herb is not an aphrodisiac, i.e. a substance to be taken at the time of sexual activity to increase virility.

(h) *Dealing with damage.* Ginseng can be used to overcome intoxication or hangover from drink, or lethargy, tiredness and poor vitality arising from drugs such as sedatives or tranquillizers, or side effects of strong medical treatment. In particular it can be used as an adjunct during chemotherapy or radiotherapy to retain some vitality and resistance. However ginseng should be used with care because it may sometimes mask a symptom that should be attended to. For example tiredness due to drug use is sometimes the result of liver damage, which should be treated accordingly.

(i) *Health in old age.* This has been dealt with fully in Chapter Seven. Suffice it to say here that for this purpose ginseng must be taken regularly — at least one course a year. The frequency of consumption should increase with age, so that after middle age some is taken every day.

——Which Kind of Ginseng Should I Take?——

This is a question that is often asked because there are so many varieties of ginseng grown in different places, there are so many products on sale, and there is a good deal of confusion between oriental *Panax ginseng,* American *Panax quinquefolium* and Russian *Eleutherococcus senticosus.* There are interesting differences in quality and usage between different varieties and species.

——————Asian ginseng (*Panax ginseng*)——————

This species is the classical ginseng about which so much has been written and researched. It is effective in all the ways discussed in this book, and is one of the most important restorative herbs in existence. It is the ideal stimulating tonic, generally more stimulating than the other species. It shouldn't be taken by people with especially nervous, hyperactive, or 'hot' disposition unless at times of exhaustion, convalescence or ageing. It is the ginseng to take if your constitution and metabolism tend to be 'cool', leading to a risk of degenerative diseases. This ginseng tends to be masculine, which means it may more successfully amplify male hormonal qualities. It therefore will be better for males to take than females, although this difference is slight and only pertains before menopause. In old age most people need the 'heat' or extra energy provided by this species.

——American ginseng (*Panax quinquefolium*)——

This species is currently available in the US and the Far East, where it is almost as popular among Orientals as the Asian species. While it does not have the same reputation of bringing life to the old and tired, it is as useful at balancing or harmonizing the metabolism, and reducing stress, as the Asian species. Moreover it is a Yin tonic, that is, it is quite suitable for people that are already highly active, energetic, nervous or choleric and wish to take ginseng for its adaptogenic activity without stoking up their fires any more. There is no difference in its male and female qualities, according to traditional sources, and can therefore be taken equally by either sex. In the Far East, American ginseng tends to be preferred in hot climates, as it is slightly cooling, whereas Asian ginseng is preferred in cold climates where it is warming.

——'Eleuthero' (*Eleutherococcus senticosus*)——

This plant, sometimes wrongly named Siberian ginseng, is somewhat like a weak ginseng. The Chinese, who call it 'ciwuja', have experience of the side by side use of this plant with true ginseng. They regard it as a mildly stimulating tonic with special qualities of restoring metabolic energy. It may be as good as ginseng in its adaptogenic effects on blood circulation and metabolism, at a much reduced price. However it does not have the restorative strength of ginseng, and will not increase vitality and well-being to anything like the same extent as Asian ginseng.

——Grades and Varieties of Ginseng Root——

It is essential to know your roots if you wish to get the best from ginseng. You cannot expect to obtain the glowing health promised in the oriental tradition from ginseng use by going into a shop and buying some cheap ginseng tablets there. I will show why below. There are many varieties and grades of root and each growing country has its own grading system. Besides, the main growing countries — China, Korea, Japan and (in the case of American ginseng only) the US, have different reputations as to quality.

Chinese ginseng

Qualities of Chinese ginseng vary from absolutely supreme quality, unavailable from any other source, down to middle quality. The very best ginseng that is available in the west is Chinese ginseng, and it is available only with difficulty, from oriental practitioners and herbal suppliers. This finest ginseng is called Yi Sun Ginseng and may cost hundreds of dollars for an ounce. It is wild ginseng transplanted into a forest bed and maintained there for several years, or partly wild ginseng grown from cultivated seed in wild conditions. A slightly lower grade is Pa-huo Tassel ginseng, which is very old ginseng, left in cultivated fields for many years — some say over 16 — after the rest of the roots are harvested. Then we have Shiu Chu ginseng, cultivated in the best possible way, and of top quality. It may be $50-$100 per ounce. The above grades are white roots, dried and sometimes preserved with sugar. Then there is Kirin ginseng, previously known as Imperial ginseng. This is simply good quality whole roots of reasonable age and size and is more commonly available. Finally we have small roots, pieces, tails etc. which go into root powder and extracts arriving in the market place in the West as capsules, tablets, teas etc. Chinese and Korean ginseng are compared as to their effects in the next section.

Korean ginseng

Korean ginseng can be excellent. The quality runs from very good roots, on the level of the Shiu Chu Chinese ginseng, down to poor material, below that of the Chinese. There may be some roots that are the result of transplanting into the wild as in the top Chinese grades, but these do not appear to be reaching the West. The top Korean grades are Korean red ginseng roots, which are classified into Heaven grade, Earth grade and Man grade. Due to government control of quality, the Koreans have managed to produce a large amount of excellent quality ginseng. As there are poorer quality imitations issuing from Hong Kong, a buyer should check that the Korean red ginseng has the seal of the 'Office of Monopoly' in Seoul, on the tins. The top grade (Heaven) Korean red ginseng roots may cost up to $50 an ounce depending on the size of the roots. The advantage of these red roots is that they are widely available all over the world and the quality is guaranteed. Korea also produces white ginseng, of middle quality, as well as the usual tails, pieces and pencil roots called Kiboshi, used to make extracts and products. John Teeguarden, an American who has made a long, practical study of Chinese tonic herbs, writes in his book *Chinese Tonic Herbs,* that Korean ginseng is 'quicker in its action and is generally more blatant' than the Chinese. 'It tones up the Yang as well as the Yin, so it will increase the fire energy, thus stimulating sexual drive and assertive, wilful behaviour. It is therefore not recommended for people with Yang, hot conditions, but is excellent for those who lack Yang energy.' Chinese ginseng tones up the Yin as much as the Yang, and it therefore may be better for long-term restorative use.

Japanese ginseng

Japanese ginseng is middle to poor in quality. There are some roots of very good quality, equivalent to the upper grades of Korean ginseng, but these do not often appear in the Western market. The majority of Japanese ginseng is poor even though it is steamed to make it red and it looks as good as Korean red roots. Indeed some Japanese roots may be very large, and those wrongly assuming size equals quality are misled. Generally, however, the poor Japanese roots find their way to Hong Kong where they reappear as imitation Korean.

How To Choose a Root

Ginseng roots are either sold singly, or packaged into boxes weighing 600 g (one 'catty'). Within each grade the roots are classified into sizes, described by the number of roots that fit into a 600 g catty. Thus an Earth grade 15 root (15 roots to the catty) is better than an Earth grade 20 root (20 roots to the catty). Though the larger the root the better it is, the grades are a more reliable indication of medicinal value than size. In other words a small root of Heaven grade Korean red ginseng is better than a large root of Earth grade.

There are some general indications of quality that are worth knowing about, besides the question of grades:

(a) *Age:* the older the root when it is harvested, the better it is.

This is probably the reason why the larger roots are more desirable within each grade.

(b) *Colour:* generally, red ginseng is better than white ginseng because only higher quality roots are selected for steaming to produce red ginseng. However there are some white roots, particularly the top grade Chinese, which are superior to red, and there are some red roots which are poor.

(c) *Density:* the root should be very hard. If it is a red root, it should be glassy or crystalline with a deep red colour.

(d) *Taste:* the taste should be rich, strong, and bitter with an edge of sweetness. If a root is tasteless, don't buy it.

(e) *Shape:* a good root is straight with intertwined rootlets or branches, sometimes giving it a man-like appearance. Curled roots are lower quality.

Roots, Extracts, Tablets and Teas

Roots are undoubtedly the best form of ginseng to take, and no ginseng cognoscenti would touch products of any kind, because they are invariably made from poor quality roots. On the other hand most people just want to take an effective, cheap, easily-taken restorative, whether it is ginseng or something else. In this case we should examine the products available, bearing in mind that none of them reaches the standard of the root.

One of the problems with products is that they are often made by western companies who do not know a great deal about ginseng, but buy in ginseng powder on the international market, and then put it into capsules or tablets. But this powder may well be very poor material to begin with and is sometimes further diluted with fillers such as lactose on its way through to the consumer. Various analytical tests have been made on ginseng products and a significant proportion of them have little or no detectable ginsenosides in them. A way round this is to choose a Korean or a Chinese product with original packaging, which is imported into the West. These will almost invariably be of better quality. If that is impossible, choose ginseng tablets or capsules from the most reputable company. In the US ginseng products now have to conform to a standard, which I helped to define, set by the Ginseng Research Institute and the National Nutritional Foods Association. Provided the system is currently in operation, only buy products which have their seal on the label.

In general it is better to buy ginseng root powder tablets or capsules than extracts, since you don't know what the extracts actually contain. However if the extracts are standardized at a certain percentage of ginsenosides, this is an indication of purity. Furthermore, thick paste extracts produced in Korea and China can be as good as any products. The product to avoid altogether is ginseng tea. You can buy ready prepared packets of instant ginseng tea, made from the root, and sometimes from the leaf or the flower of the plant. These drinks are tasty but medicinally ineffective. Today in the Far East one can buy ginseng candies, ginseng chewing gum, ginseng hair lotion, ginseng creams and cosmetics, ginseng soup flavourings and even ginseng cigarettes. Don't expect any tonic effects from these products either.

The Way to Take Ginseng

The rituals of China concerned with the consumption of ginseng are as great as those of gathering or cultivation, but almost any convenient way of ingesting it would be medically acceptable. Much of the ginseng in China is boiled and extracted for long

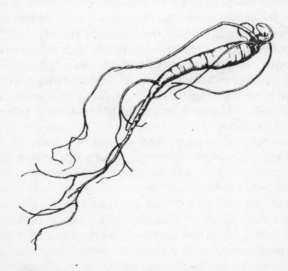

A 3-year-old ginseng root

periods with water, or water and alcohol, to give a dark extract which is sold commercially in a number of closely related forms. Drops of the extract are then taken neat or dipped into tea. Ginseng can also be chewed: a nugget of the required size is cut from the root and chewed thoroughly until it is completely soft. Another popular method is to boil the root to make a tea. Special silver kettles are used for this purpose, because it is a hard and fast rule that no other metal apart from silver can come into contact with the root. The general tradition is to boil it for between six and ten hours, starting in the evening, then get up at dawn, drink the preparation and go back to sleep. It is also common, especially among the old people, to take a whole root, together with some leaves if possible, and put it in a bottle of brandy. This is then stored for a long time, after which glasses are taken regularly with the greatest relish!

Any of these methods of consumption would be suitable for those in the West, depending on the types of root available.

How Safe is Ginseng?

It has already been mentioned that ginseng is remarkably safe, even in large doses, or when taken over a long period, and modern research has confirmed this. Professor Brekhman writes that a harmful dose for animals has been shown to be at least 1000 times the effective dose — equivalent to a man eating three to four pounds of pure ginseng at one sitting. More recently, Professor Savel of the Pharmaceutical faculty of Paris University has tried to give sufficient ginseng to mice to cause side effects. He failed: the mice suffered from enlarged stomachs due to overeating but were otherwise well.

Italian scientists gave large doses of ginseng to mice continuously for six months without any noticeable ill effects, and clinical trials with patients have never shown any harmful side effects. Health departments such as the FDA accept that ginseng is safe and allow it on open sale, without restriction.

On the other hand, it is important to realize that ginseng is, after all, a medicine, and there are no medicines known which do not have some unwanted effects under some conditions. A recent survey by an American doctor found that some people who had been taking excessive amounts of ginseng for long periods experienced various symptoms, including insomnia, over-excitation, nausea and raised blood pressure. During a trial of ginseng in the Kaschenko hospital in Russia, with some patients who were undergoing ginseng treatment for depression, 'sexual excitement was found to have been produced as a side effect.' Similar observations, including reports of a temporary return of menstruation after the menopause and of breast tenderness in elderly women, have appeared in British medical publications. A decision on whether such effects are harmful or beneficial can be left to the reader.

Ginseng is safe, but it should not be abused. The Chinese tradition states that the young and healthy do not need to take more than an occasional course of ginseng, and only the sick, debilitated and aged may take it all the time. Over-arousal can sometimes result if ginseng is taken by excitable and highly strung people, or if taken with other stimulants, such as coffee. It is recommended that for best effects, Asian ginseng should be taken in the autumn or winter rather than in the heat of the summer.

It is clear that ginseng is not toxic in itself, but that if it is taken by the right person at the right time in the right way, its effects will be maximal, and if it is taken by the wrong person at the wrong time in the wrong way its effects will be minimal or even negative. This is, of course, true of all medicines but especially the kingly Chinese remedies. In general if the reader is guided by the uses of ginseng suggested in this book, there will be little chance of any side effects.

Dosage

The label on a packet of ginseng may describe a recommended dose. How reliable are these instructions? How much of the root should one take? Are there any differences in the doses for different purposes? We can be guided in these questions by a synthesis of the Chinese traditional usage with its thousands of years experience and the careful analysis of modern science.

The Chinese chew pieces of ginseng varying in size from a pea to a walnut, and they would take more than one piece a day. This would correspond to between two and six grams of root a day, and is also the recommended dose in the *Pharmacopoeia Japonica,* but is about twice as much as is usually recommended in western preparations. This may be because the Chinese are more confident about ginseng than the Europeans. Indeed, the amounts taken by the Chinese sometimes seem to be dictated by how much they can afford rather than any other considerations. Moreover, the quality of the Chinese root is sometimes better than the root commonly available in the West, which would make the actual difference in dosage even greater. The herbal books and sources generally prescribe a dosage of approximately two grams of root a day.

We can recommend that for long-term use about one gram should be taken twice a day. However, the dose is an individual matter and each person should experiment to find the best dose for himself. A course of ginseng should last for at least a month. Older people can take ginseng continuously at a total dose of one or two grams a day. For a short-term effect, i.e. as a stimulant, to combat fatigue and exhaustion, and in cases of weakness during convalescence, the dose may be increased somewhat. Three grams a day would probably suffice, again divided into a dose in the morning and the evening. But, again, there is a correct dosage for each person, depending on factors such as constitution, need for ginseng, diet, age and state of health. It is recommended that individuals try to find the dose that is right for them by starting low and increasing the dosage until they feel they have hit the level at which they notice ginseng's positive effects.

Varying Effects

It is a common experience that some people notice the effects of ginseng and others do not. In general, most people notice a stimulation with higher doses, but this depends on whether they are exhausted or not. The more exhausted they are, the more they will notice a return to normality. During the long-term use of ginseng in lower doses, people may or may not be conscious of any change. This is because there are enormous constitutional differences in the way people respond to drugs. Thinner people, for example, tend to be more sensitive to drugs, as do those used to a simple diet. Someone on a frugal diet may notice the effects of ginseng more than someone who eats meat and rich food.

Ginseng is no more 'an alternative to pot and alcohol', as one sensation-seeking news article claims, than is garlic. On the other hand, it can undoubtedly generate a feeling of health and vitality and therefore a sense of well-being. Some people get the same feeling from a sauna bath, but it would be an exaggeration to say that a sauna bath makes people high. It can be stated categorically that there are no grounds for suggesting that ginseng has any intoxicating effect. On the contrary, it has been shown to protect the body from intoxication by alcohol and other drugs. It would thus be more accurate to say that ginseng 'helps you recover from pot and alcohol'.

CHAPTER 9 ·

Ginseng and
—Traditional Medicine—
Today

It has taken literally thousands of years for ginseng to appear in the shops in the West. Doctors are not generally familiar with it, and those who are often regard it as 'yet another useless fad'. The climate of medical opinion has hardly changed from that put forward in the Smithsonian Institute report at the beginning of the century: 'Ginseng has no value as far as western medicine can judge . . . its effects being purely psychological . . . but we have only scratched the surface of Chinese medical knowledge.'

Only a few years ago top medical experts of the West were saying exactly the same thing about acupuncture: that it had no real value, that it was mere trickery or hypnotism. They were often so scathing in their condemnation that practitioners were hardly differentiated from witches. Now the same experts have completely reversed their opinion and recognize it as a technique that has great potential usefulness. It must be said that medical experts in the West still do not understand therapeutic acupuncture at all. One might suggest that, like the apparently paradoxical aspects of ginseng, it will be hard to understand if one tries to approach it from a conventional point of view. It needs to be seen from the viewpoint of traditional medicine and the Chinese view of the body and its ailments.

—————Why Has Ginseng Been Ignored?—————

It is quite possible that ginseng will follow the same road as acupuncture. It may one day be recognized as an important new aid to health and become widely used in the West. Then the question might be raised: why is it that such an obviously beneficial substance is still not taken seriously by the medical profession? Several reasons can be suggested.

1. Many products made in western countries are of such poor quality that members of both the public and the medical profession may have begun to be interested in ginseng when it arrived, only to dismiss it when no clear effects resulted from taking one or other ginseng products.

2. Large numbers of reports have been published on ginseng in the scientific journals of China, Russia, Japan and Korea. There may be as many as 2000. Yet most of these are without translation, and very few have been read by Western scientists. This is partly because of the difficulty of getting hold of the reports, but mostly because there has been very little interest among experts for such information from the East. The flow of information on medicine and science has been mostly in one direction — from West to East. Apart from an 'information gap', there is also a 'credibility gap', so that even when some information does arrive in the West, it is often ignored or treated with suspicion, for the experts involved trust neither the authors whom they do not know, nor the journal which they do not respect.

3. Western medicines are mostly synthetic and are strictly standardized, manufactured, packaged and distributed by a large pharmaceutical industry with a powerful voice in medicine. Doctors feel that unless a medicine is of this category it should not be used. Their attitude has probably been formed by their training in medical schools, and by the advertisements of the pharmaceutical industry. The pharmaceutical industry is strongly opposed to natural medicines, because it could not support itself on the distribution of herbs and roots.

4. Ginseng, like many other herbs, has a subtle and mild effect, which is most beneficial when the root is taken regularly for a period. There is also no specific disease that can be said to be *cured* by ginseng. All the effects that have been discussed in the preceding pages are so different from conventional medicines that if comparisons are made with powerful synthetic drugs ginseng may be regarded as inconsequential. There are also some features, such as its 'adaptogenic' power, which are puzzling if regarded from a conventional point of view, although well understood in traditional medicine. Therefore, ginseng has been thought about in the past in a way

calculated to miss its most advantageous features.

────────Synthetic Drugs versus Plant Drugs────────

The strange fact is that although many doctors still do not think much of herbs and herbalism, large numbers of synthetic medicines used by doctors are originally derived from plants. The medicines may have been extracted, altered and resynthesized for the purpose of standardization and so on, but often the original discovery and isolation of the drug was made through traditional herbs: digitalis, the important heart-stabilizing glycoside from the foxglove; morphine from the poppy; quinine, once vital in the treatment of malaria, from the bark of a tree; reserpine, used in the treatment of mental disease, from raowolfia; the list is endless.

Perhaps it is not so widely known that much research is still going on to find newer and newer medicines from traditional plant remedies. Very recently, the powerful plant anti-cancer alkaloids vinblastine and vincristine were found in the plant *Vinca rosea*, which has been used since ancient times in Indian medicine. The United States' multi-million-dollar drive against cancer includes a new massive survey of medicinal plants used in traditional medicine for their possible anti-cancer properties. No one would deny that the pharmaceutical industry was founded on plants.

It would therefore be more accurate to say that the medical world is opposed to plants which have not yielded chemically defined and standardized chemicals, rather than against plants as such. As one eminent British scientist said about ginseng, 'It is no use doing any research on it until we know what it contains.' This attitude is precisely that which prevents western medical experts from understanding and utilizing the wealth of traditional medicines. Who cares what chemicals are inside the plant, as long as it works safely? There is no point in forgetting the aims of medicine in favour of extracting and synthesizing drugs.

Besides ignoring some important medicines which happen to be too complicated to yield known active ingredients, there is a more serious danger. The process of extracting and defining the active principle may leave out other constituents which are present in the plant and are important for a balanced treatment.

The herbalist understands that medicines must be as subtly balanced as music. Extraction of only one component is like throwing out all the instruments in an orchestra except the loudest. Not only is this unnecessary, it may actually be harmful. For example, aspirin was extracted from willow in the seventeenth century. It was probably the first medicine to be purified and synthesized. After 300 years of constant use, it has now been shown to cause side effects such as stomach bleeding. It would have been better not to use it in such a concentrated and purified form.

Ginseng is one of the few herbs for which there is clear scientific evidence that there are more medicinal powers in the entire plant than in any of the chemicals so far isolated from it.

There may one day be 'ginsenoside pills' available in your local pharmacy. Indeed in both the Soviet Union and Japan ginseng root material is now grown in vats in the laboratory from which a ginsenoside-rich extract is made for the pharmaceutical industry. But because of the great number of constituents, many still unknown, it is obvious that a great deal will be lost when a ginsenoside pill is made.

Multiple and Paradoxical Uses

Conventional scientific research, in attempting to extract a single chemical, also looks for a single defined action of a drug. For example, tests will be carried out to see if a drug can raise the blood pressure, or lower the blood pressure. Ginseng is unique because it seems to be one of the first herbs for which there is scientific evidence that the whole root can have multiple and apparently paradoxical effects. It can both raise and lower the blood pressure, or act as a stimulant and sedative. Allopathic medicine would prefer one defined drug to raise the blood pressure and another drug to lower it, neither of which drugs could adjust to the body's requirements as ginseng does. This shows that the very philosophy behind conventional medicine needs to be brought up to date.

It would be foolish to go to the opposite extreme and become prejudiced against conventional medicine. There are, of course, a multitude of things that the more powerful synthetic medicines can do that herbs cannot. One need only think of the new drugs available which can now eliminate tuberculosis, leprosy and malaria, or the vaccines which can completely protect a person from catching smallpox or polio or the injections which can keep a diabetic in relatively good health. My purpose is to point out that there are gaps in conventional medicine which can be very successfully filled by 'natural medicine'. Herbal medicines should be used alongside conventional medicine as in China. The herbs should be used to maintain health, as restoratives and tonics, while the stronger medicines should be used, as mentioned in the Emperor Shen Nung's *Pharmacopoeia of the Heavenly Husbandman,* when a serious illness occurs despite all the other efforts. This would be 'the best of the old and the new'.

Ginseng is being used a little more widely every day. It is already available in all health shops in the western world and is the main constituent in several geriatric preparations on sale in pharmacies. We can expect that as it gets more widely known, serious research might begin in the West on its properties. Doctors might know more about it and prescribe courses of it to increase the health of their patients, as they do in Russia and China.

In Britain, ginseng is not readily accepted by the medical profession. There is little chance that it will enter the British Pharmacopoeia in the very near future. On the other hand, there are many enthusiasts who take ginseng, including some doctors and psychiatrists. It is often in the news. Henry Kissinger, who skipped around the world with such energy, was in the news because of his possession of ginseng; so were the North Vietnamese. In fact, during the long hours of the Paris peace conference on Vietnam, the North Vietnamese delegation were never apparently tired or exhausted. When questioned about this by the other diplomats, they produced some ginseng with a flourish.

The last word should come from Sir Edwin Arnold, the famous translator, traveller and author, who eloquently sums up the case for ginseng as a result of his experience in China.

> According to the Chinese, Asiatic ginseng is the best and most potent of all cordials, stimulants, tonics, stomachics, cardiacs, febrifuges, and above all, will best renovate and invigorate failing forces. It fills the heart with hilarity, while its occasional use will, it is said, add a decade to human life. Can all these generations of Orientals who have praised heaven for ginseng's many benefits have been

totally deceived? Was humanity ever quite mistaken when half of it believed in something never puffed and never advertised?

──Further Reading──

Fulder, Stephen, *The Tao of Medicine: Ginseng, Oriental Remedies and the Pharmacology of Harmony,* Destiny Books, Rochester, Vermont (1982)

Fulder, Stephen, *An End To Ageing?,* Thorsons, Wellingborough, Northamptonshire (1983)

Tierra, Michael, *The Way of Herbs,* Washington Square Press, Simon and Shuster, New York (1983)

Teeguarden, Ron, *Chinese Tonic Herbs,* Japan Publications, Tokyo and New York (1984)

Harding, A. R., *Ginseng and Other Medicinal Plants,* facsimile of the original 1908 edition published by Emporium Publications, Boston, Mass. (1972)

Harriman, Sarah, *The Book of Ginseng,* Pyramid Books, New York (1975)

Hyatt, Richard, *Chinese Herbal Medicine,* Thorsons, Wellingborough, Northamptonshire (1984)

Kaptchuk, Ted, *The Web That Has No Weaver, Understanding Chinese Medicine,* St Martins Press, New York (1984)

Hsu, Dr Hong-Yen, and Peacher, Dr William G., *Chinese Medicine and Herb Therapy,* Oriental Healing Arts Institute, Los Angeles (1982)

Ginseng Research Institute, *Indexed Bibliography of Scientific Literature,* Roxbury, New York (1986)

──Useful research summaries are:──

Court, W. E., 'Ginseng — a Chinese Folk Medicine of Current Interest', *Pharmaceutical Journal,* 214, 180-1 (1973)

Brekhman, I. I. and Dardymov, I. V., 'New Substances of Plant Origin Which Increase Nonspecific Resistance', *Annual Review of Pharmacology,* 9, 419-430 (1969)

Phillipson, J. D. and Anderson, L. A., 'Ginseng — Quality, Safety and Efficacy?', *Pharmaceutical Journal,* 232, 161-165 (1984)

Owen, R. T., 'Ginseng: a Pharmacological Profile', *Drugs of Today,* 18, 343-351 (1981)

Index